Maylis de Kerangal

MEND THE LIVING

Translated from the French by Jessica Moore

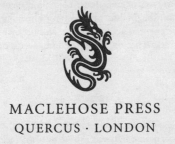

MACLEHOSE PRESS
QUERCUS · LONDON

First published in the French language as *Réparer les vivants* by
Editions Gallimard, Paris, 2014
First published in Great Britain in 2016 by MacLehose Press
This paperback edition published in 2016 by

MacLehose Press
An imprint of Quercus Publishing Ltd
Carmelite House
50 Victoria Embankment
London EC4Y 0DZ

An Hachette UK company

A CIP catalogue record for this book is available
from the British Library.

ISBN (MMP) 978 0 85705 385 5
ISBN (Ebook) 978 0 85705 386 2

10 9 8 7 6 5 4 3

Designed and typeset in Minion by Libanus Press
Printed and bound in Great Britain by Clays Ltd, St Ives plc

"My heart is full."

Paul Newman

in *The Effect of Gamma Rays on Man-in-the-Moon Marigolds* (1972)

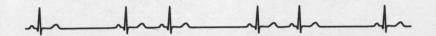

WHAT IT IS, SIMON LIMBEAU'S HEART, THIS HUMAN HEART,
from the moment of birth when its cadence accelerated while other
hearts outside were accelerating too, hailing the event, no one really
knows; what it is, this heart, what has made it leap, swell, sicken, waltz
light as a feather or weigh heavy as a stone, what has stunned it, what
has made it melt – love; what it is, Simon Limbeau's heart, what it has
filtered, recorded, archived, black box of a twenty-year-old body –
only a moving image created by ultrasound could echo it, could show
the joy that dilates and the sorrow that constricts, only the paper
printout of an electrocardiogram, unrolled from the very beginning,
could trace the form, could describe the exertion and the effort, the
emotion that rushes through, the energy required to compress itself
nearly a hundred thousand times every day and to circulate up to five
litres of blood each minute, only this could sketch the life – life of
ebbs and flows, life of valves and flapgates, life of pulsations; and
when Simon Limbeau's heart, this human heart, slips from the grip of
the machines, no one could claim to know it; and on this night – a
night without stars – while it was bone-crackingly cold on the estuary
and in the Caux region, while a reflectionless swell rolled along the
base of the cliffs, while the continental plateau drew back, unveiling

its geological stripes, this heart was sounding the regular rhythm of an organ at rest, a muscle slowly recharging – a pulse of probably less than fifty beats per minute – when a mobile phone alarm went off at the foot of a narrow bed, the echo of a sonar inscribing the digits 5.50 a.m. in luminescent bars on the touchscreen, and everything suddenly shot ahead.

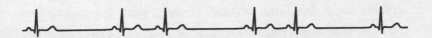

ON THIS NIGHT, THEN, A VAN SLOWS IN A DESERTED PARKING lot, comes to a crooked stop, front doors slamming while a side door slides open, three figures emerge, three shadows cut out against the dark and seized by the cold – glacial February, liquid rhinitis, sleep with your clothes on – boys, it looks like, who zip their jackets up to their chins, unroll their hats down to their eyebrows, slip the bare tips of their ears under the polar fleece and, blowing into cupped hands, turn toward the sea, which is no more than sound at this hour, sound and darkness.

Boys, now it's clear. They stand side by side behind the low wall that separates the parking lot from the beach, pacing and breathing hard, nostrils inflamed from piping iodine and cold, and they probe this dark stretch where there is no tempo besides the roar of the wave exploding, this din that swells in the final collapse, they scan what thunders before them, this mad clamour where there's nothing to rest your eyes upon, nothing, except perhaps the whitish, foaming edge, billions of atoms catapulted one against the other in a phosphores- cent halo, and, struck dumb by winter when they'd stepped out of the van, stunned by the marine night, the three boys get hold of themselves now, adjust their vision, their hearing, evaluate what awaits them, the swell, gauge it by ear, estimate its breaker index, its coefficient of depth, and remember that bluewater waves always move faster than the fastest speedboats.

Alright, one of the three boys whispers, this is gonna be awesome, the other two smile, then all three of them back up together, slowly, scraping the ground with the soles of their shoes and circling like tigers, they lift their eyes to bore into the night at the end of the village, the night still sealed shut behind the cliffs, and then the one who spoke first looks at his watch, another fifteen minutes, guys, and they get back into the van to await the nautical dawn.

Christophe Alba, Johan Rocher, and him, Simon Limbeau. The alarms were ringing when they pushed back the sheets and got out of bed for a session planned by text a little before midnight, a session at half-tide, only two or three like this a year – rough sea, regular waves, low wind, and not a soul in sight. Jeans, shirt, they slipped outside without a bite, not even a glass of milk or handful of cereal, not even a crust of bread, stood outside their building (Simon), stepped out the doorway of their suburban house (Johan), and waited for the van (Chris) that was just as punctual as they were, and the three of them who never got up before noon on Sunday, despite any and all maternal summons, the three of them who, they say, don't know how to do anything but pendulate, wet noodles, between living-room couch and bedroom armchair, these same three were chattering in the street at six in the morning, laces loose and breath rank – under the streetlight, Simon Limbeau watched the air he exhaled disintegrate, the metamorphosis of gas and smoke that lifted, compact, and dissolved into the atmosphere until it disappeared completely, remembered that when he was a kid he liked to pretend he was smoking, would hold his index and middle finger stiff in front of his lips, take a deep inhale, hollowing out his cheeks, and blow out like a man – the three of them, that is, *The Three Caballeros*, the *Big Wave Riders*, namely Chris, John and Sky, aliases that act not as nicknames but rather as pseudonyms, created in order to reinvent themselves, planetary surfers, when really they're high-schoolers from the estuary, so that saying their real first names pushes them back immediately into a hostile configuration, back to icy drizzle, feeble lapping, cliffs like walls, and streets deserted as evening falls, parental reproach and school's summonses, complaints from the girlfriend left behind, the one who, once again, came second place to the *van*, the one who is powerless when it comes to surfing.

They're in the van – they never say it in French, *camionnette*, would rather die. Dank humidity, sand granulating surfaces and scraping butts like a scouring pad, brackish rubber, stench of paraffin and the beach, surfboards piled up, heap of wetsuits – shorties or thick steamers with built-in hoods – gloves, boots, bars of wax, leashes. Sitting down all together in the front, squeezed in shoulder to shoulder, rubbed their hands together between their thighs letting out monkey yelps, it's fucking freezing, and then munched on energy bars – but they couldn't peck it all down, it's afterwards that you devour, after you've been devoured yourself – passed the bottle of Coke back and forth, the tube of Nestlé condensed milk, the Pepitos and the Chamonix, soft sugary cookies for soft sugary boys, finally pulled the latest issue of *Surf Session* out from under the seat and opened it on the dashboard, leaning their three heads together above the pages that gleam in the half-light, glossy paper like skin rubbed with suntan lotion and pleasure, pages turned thousands of times before that they pore over again now, eyeballs tumbling out of their sockets, mouths dry: giants at Mavericks and point breaks in Lombok, Jaws in Hawaii, tubes at Vanuatu, swells at Margaret River – the best coastlines on the planet roll out the splendour of surfing before their eyes. They point at images with a fervent index, there, there, they'll go there one day, maybe even next summer, the three of them in the van for a legendary surf trip, they'll go in search of the most beautiful wave that's ever formed on earth, they'll set off in pursuit of that wild and secret spot they'll invent just as Christopher Columbus invented America and they'll be alone on the line-up when it finally emerges, the one they've been waiting for, this wave risen from the bottom of the ocean, archaic and perfect, beauty personified, and the motion and the speed will stand them up on their boards in a rush of adrenalin while over their whole bodies right to the tips of their lashes will pearl a terrible joy, and they'll mount the wave, joining the earth and the tribe of surfers, this nomadic humanity with hair discoloured by salt and eternal summer, with washed-out eyes, boys and girls with nothing else to wear but shorts printed with gardenias or hibiscus petals, turquoise or blood-orange T-shirts, with no shoes other than those plastic flip-flops, these youths polished by sun and freedom: they'll surf the fold all the way to shore.

The pages of the magazine brighten as the sky pales outside, divulge their colour chart of blues, like this pure cobalt that assaults the eyes, and greens so deep you'd think they were painted in acrylic, here and there the wake of a surfboard appears, tiny white line on the phenomenal wall of water, the boys blink, murmur, that shit is epic, that's sick, then Chris shifts to check his phone, the screen illuminates him from below and turns his face blue, accentuates the bone structure – prominent brow, prognathous jaw, mauve lips – while he reads the day's forecast out loud: Petites-Dalles today, ideal northeast swell, waves between one metre fifty and one metre eighty, best session of the year; and then he punctuates, ceremonious: we're gonna pig out, *yesss*, we're gonna be *kings!* – English embedded in their French constantly, for everything and nothing, English as though they were living in a pop song or an American sitcom, as though they were heroes, foreigners, English that makes enormous words breezy, "*vie*" and "*amour*" becoming the offhanded "life" and "love", and finally English like a show of reserve – and John and Sky nod their heads in a sign of infinite agreement, yeah, big wave riders, kings.

It's time. Beginning of the day when the shapeless takes shape: the elements gather, the sky separates from the sea, the horizon grows clear. The three boys get ready, methodical, following a precise order that is still a ritual: they wax their boards, check the leashes are attached, slip into thermal rash guards before pulling on their suits, contorting themselves in the parking lot – neoprene adheres to the skin, scrapes and even burns it sometimes – choreography of rubber puppets who ask each other for help, requiring that they touch and manipulate each other; and then the surf boots, the hood, the gloves, and they close the van. They walk down toward the ocean, surfboard under one arm, light, cross the beach in long strides, the beach where pebbles crash beneath their feet in an infernal racket, and once they've arrived at water's edge, while everything grows clear before them, the chaos and the party, they each wrap a leash around an ankle, adjust their hoods, reduce the space of bare skin around their necks to nothing by grabbing the cords at their backs and pulling them up to the last notch of the zipper – it's a matter of ensuring the best possible degree of waterproofness for their teenage-boy skin, skin that's often studded with acne on the upper back, on the shoulder blades, where Simon Limbeau sports a Maori tattoo as a pauldron – and this movement, arm extended sharply, signifies that the session is starting, let's go! And maybe now, hearts get worked up, maybe they shake themselves inside thoracic cages, maybe their mass and their volume augment and their kick intensifies, two distinct sequences in one same pulsing, two beats, always the same: terror and desire.

They enter the water. Don't yell as they dive in, squeezed inside this flexible membrane that guards body heat and the explosiveness of the rush, don't emit a single cry, only grimace as they cross the low wall of rolling pebbles, and the sea gets deep fast – five or six metres out they already can't touch bottom, they topple forward, stretching themselves out flat on their boards, and with arms strongly notching the wave, they cross the breakwater and move out toward the open.

Two hundred metres from shore, the sea is no more than an undulating tautness – it grows hollow and swells up, lifted like a sheet thrown over a mattress. Simon Limbeau melts into his movement, paddles toward the line-up, that zone in the open where the surfer waits for the wave, checking that Chris and John are there, little black barely visible floats off to the left. The water is dark, marbled, veined, the colour of tin. Still no shine, no sparkle, just these white particles that powder the surface, sugar, and the water is freezing, nine or ten degrees Celsius, no more, Simon won't be able to ride more than nine or ten waves, he knows it, surfing in cold water exhausts the organism, in an hour he'll be cooked, he has to select, choose the wave with the best shape, the one whose crest will be high but not too pointed, the one whose curl will open with enough breadth for him to enter,

14

the one that will last all the way, conserving enough force to churn up on to the shore.

He turns back toward the coast, as he always likes to before going farther: the earth is there, stretched out, black crust in the bluish glow, and it's another world, a world he's unlinked to now. The cliff, a standing sagittal slice, shows him the strata of time, but out here where he is, there is no time, there's no history, only this unpredictable flow that carries and swirls him. His gaze lingers on the vehicle decked out like a Californian van in the parking lot beside the beach – he recognises the side studded with stickers, collected over many surf trips, he knows the names clustered shoulder-to-shoulder, Rip Curl, Oxbow, Quiksilver, O'Neill, Billabong, the psychedelic fresco mixing surfing champions and rock stars in the same bedazzled jumble, including a good number of girls with backs arched in itsy-bitsy bikinis, with mermaid hair, this van that is their communal artwork and the antechamber of the wave – and then he follows the tail lights of a car that climbs the plateau and plunges into the interior, Juliette's sleeping profile traces itself, she's lying curled up under her little-girl blanket, she has the same stubborn look even when she's asleep, and suddenly he turns, away from the continent, tears himself from it with a jerk, a few dozen metres more, then he stops paddling.

Arms that rest but legs that steer, hands holding the rails of the board and chest slightly raised, chin high, Simon Limbeau floats. He waits. Everything around him is in flux – whole sections of sea and sky emerge and disappear with each swirl of the slow, heavy, ligneous surface, a basaltic batter. The abrasive dawn burns his face and his skin stretches taut, his eyelashes harden like vinyl threads, the lenses behind his pupils frost over as though they'd been forgotten in the back of a freezer and his heart begins to slow, responding to the cold, when suddenly he sees it coming, he sees it moving forward, firm and

15

homogenous, the wave, the promise, and he instinctively positions himself to find the entrance and flow into it, slide in like a bandit slides his hand into a treasure chest to rob the loot – same hood, same millimetred precision of the movement – to slip on to the back of the wave, in this torsion of matter where the inside proves itself to be more vast and more profound than the outside, it's here, thirty metres away, it's coming at a constant speed, and suddenly, concentrating his energy in his shoulders, Simon launches himself and paddles with all his might so he can catch the wave with speed, so he can be taken by its slope, and now it's the *take-off*, superfast phase when the whole world concentrates and rushes forward, temporal flash when you have to inhale sharply, hold your breath and gather your body into a single action, give it the vertical momentum that will stand it up on the board, feet planted wide, left one in front, *regular*, legs bent, and back flat nearly parallel to the board, arms spread to stabilise it all, and this second is decidedly Simon's favourite, the one that allows him to grasp the whole explosion of his own existence, and to conciliate himself with the elements, to integrate himself into the living, and once he's standing on the board – estimated height from trough to crest at that moment is over one metre fifty – to stretch out space, lengthen time, and until the end of the run to exhaust the energy of each atom in the sea. Become the unfurling, become the wave.

He lets out a whoop as he takes this first ride, and for a period of time he touches a state of grace – it's horizontal vertigo, he's neck and neck with the world, and as though issued from it, taken into its flow – space swallows him, crushes him as it liberates him, saturates his muscular fibres, his bronchial tubes, oxygenates his blood; the wave unfolds on a blurred timeline, slow or fast it's impossible to tell, it suspends each second one by one until it finishes pulverised, an organic, senseless mess and it's incredible but after having been battered by pebbles in the froth at the end, Simon Limbeau turns to go straight back out again, without even touching down, without even stopping to look at the fleeting shapes that form in the foam when the sea stumbles over the earth, surface against surface, he turns back toward the open, paddling even harder now, ploughing toward that threshold where everything begins, where everything is stirred up, he joins his two friends who would soon let out that same cry in the descent, and the set of waves that comes tearing down upon them from the horizon, bleeding their bodies dry, gives them no respite.

No other surfer comes to join them at the spot, no one approaches the parapet to watch them surf nor sees them come out of the water an hour later, spent, done in, knees like jelly, stumbling across the beach to the parking lot and opening the doors of the van, no one sees their feet and their hands the same shade of blue, bruised, purpled even beneath the nails, nor the abrasions that lacerate their faces now, the chapping at the corners of their lips as their teeth clatter clack clack clack, a continuous trembling of the jaws in time with the uncontainable shaking of their bodies; no one sees anything, and when they're dressed again, wool long johns under their jeans, layers of sweaters, leather gloves, no one sees them rubbing one another's backs, unable to say anything but holy shit, holy fuck, when they would have so liked to talk, to describe the rides, write the legend of the session, and shivering like that, they get in the van and close the door, without pausing for even a second Chris finds the strength to put the key in the ignition, he starts the car and off they go.

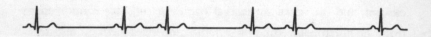

IT'S CHRIS WHO DRIVES — IT'S ALWAYS HIM, THE VAN BELONGS to his father and neither Johan nor Simon has their licence. From Petites-Dalles it's about an hour to Le Havre if you take the old road from Étretat that goes down the estuary through Octeville-sur-Mer, the Ignauval Valley and Sainte-Adresse.

The boys have stopped shivering, the heat in the van is on full blast, the music too, and probably the sudden warmth inside is another thermal shock for them, probably fatigue catches up now, they probably yawn, heads nodding, trying to nestle against the back of the seats, swaddled and soothed inside the vehicle's vibrations, noses tucked snug into their scarves, and probably they also grow numb, eyelids closing intermittently, and maybe, when they passed Étretat, Chris accelerated without even realising it, shoulders slumped, hands heavy on the wheel, the road straight ahead now, yes, maybe he said to himself it's okay, the road's clear, and the desire to make the return journey go faster so they could get home and stretch out, re-enter reality after the session, its violence, maybe this desire ended up weighing on the gas pedal, so that he let himself go, carving through the plateau and the black fields, soil turned over, the fields somnolent too, and maybe the perspective of the highway — an arrowhead thrusting forward before the windshield as on a video game screen – ended up hypnotising him like a mirage, so that he lashed himself to it, let go his vigilance, and everyone remembers there was a frost that night, winter dusting the landscape like parchment paper, everyone knows about the patches of black ice on the pavement, invisible beneath the dull sky but inking out the roadsides, and everyone imagines the patches of fog that float at irregular intervals, compact, water evaporating from the mud at the rate of the rising day, dangerous pockets that filter the outside and erase every landmark, yes, okay, and what else, what more? An animal in the road? A lost cow, a dog that crawled under a fence, a fox with a fiery tail or even a sudden human shape, ghostly at the edge of the embankment, that had to be avoided at the last second with a jerk of the wheel? Or a song? Yes, maybe the girls in bikinis who adorned the body of the van suddenly came to life and crawled up over the hood, overtaking the windshield, lascivious, their green hair tumbling down, and unloosing their inhuman (or too human) voices, and maybe Chris lost his head, sucked into their trap, hearing this singing that was not of this world, the song of the sirens, the song that kills? Or maybe Chris just made a wrong move, yes, that's it, like the tennis player misses an easy shot, like the skier catches an edge, one dumb mistake, maybe he didn't turn the wheel when the road was turning, or, finally, because this hypothesis also has to be made, maybe Chris fell asleep at the wheel, leaving the stark countryside to enter the tube of a wave, the marvellous and suddenly intelligible spiral that stretched out before his surfboard, siphoning the world with it, the world and all of its blue.

Emergency medical services arrived at the scene around 9.20 a.m. – ambulances, police – and signs were set out to detour traffic on to smaller collateral roads and protect the accident scene. The most important thing had been to get the three boys' bodies out, imprisoned inside the vehicle, tangled with those of the mermaid girls who smiled on the hood, or winced, deformed, crushed one against the other, shreds of thighs, buttocks, breasts.   —

They could easily determine that the little van was going fast, they estimated its speed at ninety-two kilometres an hour, which was twenty-two kilometres an hour over the speed limit for this section of road, and they also determined that, for unknown reasons, it had drifted over to the left without ever coming back into its lane, hadn't braked – no tyre marks on the asphalt – and that it had crashed into this pole at full force; they noted the absence of airbags, the van model was too old, and they could see that of the three passengers seated in the front, only two were wearing seat belts – one on each side, the driver's and the passenger's; finally, they determined that the third individual, sitting in the middle, had been propelled forward by the violence of the impact, head hitting the windshield; it had taken twenty minutes to pull him from the metal, unconscious when the ambulances arrived, heart still beating, and, having found his cafeteria card in the pocket of his jacket, they determined that his name was Simon Limbeau.

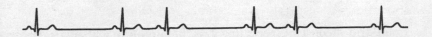

PIERRE REVOL STARTED HIS SHIFT AT EIGHT THIS MORNING. HE scanned his magnetic card at the entrance to the parking lot while the night turned greyscale – pale, still sky, vaguely turtledove, a far cry in any case from the grandiloquent choreographies that had given the clouds of the estuary their pictorial reputation – drove slowly across the hospital grounds, snaking between buildings that were connected according to a complex plan, slid into the place reserved for him, parked his car nose first, a petroleum-blue Laguna, a vehicle in decline but still comfortable, leather interior and good radio, the preferred model of taxi barons he says with a smile, then he went into the hospital, crossed the enormous windowed nave toward the north hall, ground floor, and, walking fast, arrived at the hyperbaric medicine and intensive care unit.

He passes through the department door, pushing it open with the flat of his hand so firmly that it bangs several times in the emptiness after him, and those who are at the end of the night shift, men and women in white or green shirts, all of them done in, dishevelled, brisk movements and bright eyes, febrile grins on their tense faces – tambourine skin – these ones laughing too loudly, or coughing, frog in their throats, voiceless, these ones bump into him in the corridor, brush past him or on the contrary see him coming from far off, cast a glance at their watches and bite their lips, think, good, finally, in ten minutes I can get out of here, in ten minutes I'm off, and at that moment their features relax, change colour, turn pallid, and circles trace themselves all at once, bronze spoons beneath their blinking eyelids.

Calm strides, constant speed, Revol reaches his office without deviating from his path to respond to this sign someone is already making, these papers someone is already holding out, this intern who's already hot on his heels; takes his key out in front of an ordinary door, enters, and proceeds to the daily gestures of arriving at work: hangs his coat – a tan trench coat – on the peg nailed to the back of the door, pulls on his white coat, turns on the coffee maker, the computer, absently taps the paperwork that plasters his desk, surveys the stack, sits down, connects to the internet, sorts the messages in his inbox, writes one or two replies – no hello or anything, all words emptied of their vowels and no punctuation – then gets up and takes a deep breath. He's in good shape, he's feeling good.

He's a tall man, skinny, thorax hollowed and belly round – solitude – long arms long legs, white leather lace-ups, something slender and uncertain in him that matches his juvenile mien, and his coat is always open, so that when he moves the panels swell, spread, wings, revealing jeans and a shirt, also white, and rumpled.

The little diode glows at the base of the coffee maker while the bitter scent of the electric hotplate heating empty fills the air, the dregs of coffee cool in the glass pot. Although minuscule – five or six lousy square metres – this private space is a privilege at the hospital and so it's surprising to find it this impersonal, chaotic, of a questionable cleanliness: swivelling chair that's comfortable despite the high seat, desk where forms of all sorts pile up, along with papers, notebooks, notepads, and promotional pens palmed off by laboratories in plastic embossed pouches, a bottle of San Pellegrino gone flat and, in a frame, photo of a Mont Aigoual landscape; punctuating the clutter, three objects placed in an isosceles triangle may testify to an urge to add a personal touch – a glass paperweight from Venice, a stone turtle, and a cup for pencils; against the back wall, a metal shelf holds disparate folders and boxes of files numbered by year, a good layer of dust, and a small handful of books whose titles you can read if you get closer: the two tomes of *The Hour of Our Death* by Philippe Ariès, *La sculpture du vivant* by Jean Claude Ameisen from the Points Sciences collection, a book by Margaret Lock with a two-tone cover illustrating a brain called *Twice Dead: Organ Transplants and the Reinvention of Death*, an issue of the *Neurological Review* from 1959, and the crime novel by Mary Higgins Clark *Moonlight Becomes You* – a book Revol likes, we'll find out why later. Otherwise no window, hard fluorescent, the bare light of a kitchen at three in the morning.

Within the hospital, the I.C.U. is a separate space that takes in tangential lives, opaque comas, deaths foretold – it houses these bodies situated exactly at the point between life and death. A domain of hallways and rooms where suspense holds sway. Revol performs here, on the reverse side of the diurnal world, the world of continuing, stable life, of days that irrupt in the light and file toward future plans, he works in the hollow of this territory the way you'd rummage inside a heavy coat, inside its dark folds, its cavities. And he likes his shifts,

Sundays and nights, has liked them since his residency – you can imagine Revol as a slender young intern seduced by the very idea of the job, this feeling of being needed, at work and autonomous, called upon to ensure the continuity of the medical gesture within a given perimeter, invested with vigilance and endowed with a responsibility. He likes their alveolar intensity, their specific temporality, fatigue like a surreptitious stimulant that gradually rises through the body, accelerates and makes it sharper, all this erotic turmoil; likes their vibratile silence, their half-light – devices that blink in the dimness, blue computer screens or desk lamps like the flame of a candle in a La Tour painting – *The Newborn*, for example – and again this physicality of the work, this climate of an enclave, this watertightness, the department like a spaceship launched into a black hole, a submarine plunging into a bottomless chasm, The Mariana Trench. But Revol has been getting something else from this work for a long time: the stark consciousness of his own existence. Not a feeling of power, not a megalomaniac exultation – exactly the opposite: an influx of lucidity that regulates his movements and sifts his decisions. A shot of cold-blood.

Department meeting: the transmittals. The staff from both shifts are here, they form a circle, everyone stays standing, leaning against the walls with cups in hand. The team leader, who oversaw the previous shift, is a thirty-year-old fellow, sturdy, with thick hair and muscled arms. Exhausted, he glows. Details the situation of the patients present in the unit – for example, the absence of any notable change in the eighty-four-year-old man, still unconscious after sixty days of intensive care, whereas the neurological status of that young woman, admitted two months ago after an overdose, has declined – before giving a longer description of the newly admitted patients: a fifty-seven-year-old woman with no fixed address, advanced cirrhosis, admitted after having convulsions at the shelter, remains haemodynamically unstable; a forty-year-old man, admitted that evening after a heart attack, with cerebral oedema – a jogger, he was running on the seafront toward Cape de la Hève, luxury cross-trainers on his feet, head encircled with a neon orange bandana, when he collapsed near the Café de l'Estacade, and, even though they wrapped him in a thermal blanket, he was blue when admitted, soaked in sweat, features hollow. Where are we at with him? Revol asks in a neutral tone, leaning against the window. A nurse answers, specifies that the vitals (pulse rate, blood pressure, body temperature, respiration rate) are normal, urine output is low, the P.I.V. (peripheral intravenous line) has been placed. Revol doesn't know this woman, inquires about the patient's blood test results, she answers that they are in process. Revol looks at his watch, okay, we're good to go. The team disperses.

This same nurse lingers in the room, intercepts Revol and holds out her hand: Cordelia Owl, I'm new, I was in the O.R. before. Revol nods, okay, welcome – if he had looked more closely, he would have seen that there was something a little odd about her, eyes clear but marks on her neck, swollen lips, knots in her hair, bruises on her knees, he might wonder where this floating smile came from, this Mona Lisa smile that doesn't leave even when she leans over patients to clean their eyes and mouths, inserts breathing tubes, checks vital signs, administers treatments, and maybe if he did he would be able to guess that she had seen her lover again last night, that he had phoned her after weeks of silence, the dog, and that she showed up on an empty stomach, beauteous, decorated like a reliquary, lids smoky, hair shining, breasts warm, resolved to an amicable distance, but she was a rather mezzo actor, whispering distantly how are you? it's good to see you, while inside her whole body was diffusing its turmoil, incubating its tumult, a hot ember, so they drank one beer and then two, attempted conversations that didn't take, and then she went outside to smoke, telling herself over and over I should go now, I should go this is stupid, but he came outside to find her, I'm not gonna stay long, I don't want to be up too late, a feint, and then he got out his lighter to light her cigarette, she sheltered the flame with her hands, tilting her head, curls falling across her face and threatening to become a wick, he tucked them automatically behind her ear again, the pads of his fingers brushing her temple, so automatically that she went weak, the backs of her knees turning to jelly – all of this, by the way, threadbare and old as the hills – and bang, a few seconds later the two of them were knocking about beneath a neighbouring porch, held inside the darkness and the smell of cheap wine, banging into garbage cans, offering a range of pale skin, upper thighs emerging from jeans or tights, bellies appearing beneath lifted shirts or unbuckled belts, buttocks, everything boiling and freezing all at once as their mutual and violent desire collides – yes, if Revol looked at her more closely, he would see in Cordelia Owl a girl who was curiously bright-eyed, even though she was beginning her shift on a sleepless night, a girl in much better shape than he was, someone he would be able to count on.

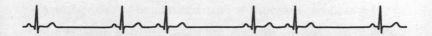

WE HAVE SOMEONE FOR YOU. A CALL AT 10.12 A.M. NEUTRAL, informative, the words strike. Male, six feet, 154 pounds, about twenty years old, car accident, head trauma, in a coma – we know who's being summed up like this, we know his name: Simon Limbeau. The call is barely finished when the ambulance crew arrives, the fireproof doors open, the stretcher rolls in, up the central hallway of the I.C.U., people step aside to let it pass. Revol emerges – he's just been to examine the patient admitted in the night after convulsions, and he's not optimistic: the woman didn't receive C.P.R. in time, the scanner revealed that liver cells had died after her heart stopped, a sign that her brain cells were also affected – he'd been put on alert, and, seeing the trolley arrive at the end of the hallway, he suddenly says to himself that this Sunday's shift won't be easy.

The doctor from emergency services follows the stretcher. He's built like a high alpine surveyor, bald, mid-fifties, skin and bone, a twig; he reveals pointy teeth when he says out loud: Glasgow 3! Then addresses himself specifically to Revol: the neurological exams showed a lack of response to sound (calling his name), visual stimuli (light), or pain; there were also ocular disturbances (asymmetrical movements of the eyes), and respiratory dysfunctions; they had

27

intubated him immediately. He closes his eyes, rubbing his head from forehead toward the occiput: suspected cerebral haemorrhaging following head trauma, unresponsive coma, Glasgow 3 – he uses this language they share, language that banishes the verbose as a waste of time, exiles eloquence and the seduction of words, overdoes nouns, codes and acronyms, language in which to speak signifies above all to describe – in other words, inform a team, gather up all the evidence in order to allow a diagnosis to be made, tests to be ordered, to allow people to treat and to save: power of the succinct. Revol takes in each piece of information, and plans for the body scan.

Cordelia Owl is the one who sets him up in his room, in his bed, after which the E.S. team can leave the department, taking their equipment with them – stretcher, portable ventilator, oxygen tank. Now they have to insert an arterial line, electrodes on his chest, a urinary catheter, and connect Simon to the monitors that will show his vital signs – lines of different colours and forms appear, superposed, straight or broken lines, cross-hatched deviations, rhythmic undulations: the Morse code of medicine. Cordelia works with Revol, her gestures are assured, her movements fluid, easy, her body seems relieved of the viscous spleen that still clung to her movements only yesterday.

An hour later, death shows up, death announces itself, a moving spot with an irregular circumference opacifying a shape that is lighter and more vast, here it is, it's arrived. Vision sharp as a cudgel blow but Revol doesn't blink, concentrating on the shots of the body scan on his computer screen, labyrinthine images with legends like geographical maps that he rotates in all directions and zooms in on, getting his bearings, measuring the distances, while on his desk, within arm's reach, a folder with the hospital's logo contains a paper copy of the images considered "relevant", provided by the medical imaging department where Simon Limbeau's brain was scanned – his head was swept by X-rays to produce these images, and, according to what's called electron tomography, the data was seized by "slice", "cuts" of a millimetre thick that could be analysed on all planes of space, coronal, axial, sagittal and oblique. Revol knows how to read these images and what they confirm in terms of the state of the subject, what they herald in terms of developments; he recognises these shapes, these spots, these halos, interprets these milky rings, decrypts these black marks, deciphers legends and codes; he compares, verifies, starts again, carries out his investigation all the way to the end, but there's nothing to be done, it's already over: Simon Limbeau's brain is on the verge of destruction – it's drowning in blood.

Diffuse lesions, severe cerebral swelling, and nothing that could keep the intracranial pressure under control, it's already much too high. Revol sinks back in his chair. His hand comes to cup his chin as his gaze trails across the desk, skims over the disorder, the scribbled notes, the administrative circulars, the photocopy of an article issued by the ethics committee of the Paris public hospital administration on organ recovery "after the heart has stopped"; his eyes glide over the small objects placed there, including the turtle carved of jade, a present from a young patient with severe asthma, grind to a halt on the mauve slopes of Mount Aigoual draped in streaming run-off and Revol probably thinks back, then, in a flash, to that day in September when he was initiated into peyote at his house in Vallerauge – Marcel and Sally arrived at the end of the afternoon in an emerald-green sedan, the rims splattered with dried mud, the vehicle stopped heavily in the courtyard, and Sally waved her hand out the window yoo-hoo we're here! her snowy-white hair flying about inside the car, revealing her wooden earrings, duo of varnished scarlet cherries; later, after dinner, when night had fallen over the plateau, a shower of bright stars, they went out into the garden and Marcel's hands pulled back a newspaper wrapping to reveal a few small verdigris cacti, round and without spines; the three friends rolled in their palms and breathed in the bitter smell; these fruits came from far away, Marcel and Sally had gone to get them in a mining desert in northern Mexico, illegally stowed and carefully transported them all the way to the Cévennes, and Pierre, who studied hallucinogenic plants, was impatient to try it: he was fascinated by the idea of these visions from nowhere, brought on by the combination of powerful alkaloids contained in peyote, one-third mescaline, visions with no link to memory – visions that played a major role in the ritual use of this cactus, usually consumed by native Americans during shamanic ceremonies. Even more, Pierre was interested in the synesthesia that sometimes happened during hallucinations: psychosensory alertness was supposed to be most intense in the first phase after ingestion, and he hoped to see tastes, see odours, see sounds and tactile sensations, and hoped that the translation of senses into images would help him to understand – to pierce – the mystery of pain. Revol thinks back to that sparkling night, when the canopy of heaven tore open over the mountains, revealing unsuspected spaces into which they attempted to dive, lying in the grass with their backs to the earth, and suddenly he's struck by the idea of a universe in expansion, in a state of perpetual becoming, a space where cellular death would be the catalyst for metamorphosis, where death would shape the living the way silence shapes sound, darkness the light, or static the mobile; a fleeting intuition that persists on his retina even now when his eyes come back to skim over his computer screen, this sixteen-inch rectangle radiated by black light announcing the cessation of all mental activity in Simon Limbeau's brain. He's not able to connect the young man's face with death, and his throat grows tight. Nearly thirty years, though, that he's been working in death's vicinity, thirty years that he's been hanging around the sector.

Pierre Revol was born in 1959. Cold War, triumph of the Cuban revolution, first vote for Swiss women in the canton of Vaud, filming of Godard's *Breathless*, release of Burroughs's *Naked Lunch* and Miles Davis's mythical opus, *Kind of Blue* – only the most important jazz album of all time, to quote Revol, who likes to show off, lauding the vintage quality of his birth year. Anything else? Yes – he adopts a detached tone, crafting his delivery carefully (we imagine him avoiding the gaze of his interlocutor and doing everything else possible, digging in his pocket, punching in a number on his phone, deciphering a message) – it was also the year they redefined death. And at that moment, he's rather pleased with the mix of astonishment and fear he glimpses on the faces of those around him. Lifting his head and smiling vaguely, he adds: which, for an intensive care anaesthetist, is hardly insignificant.

In fact, in 1959, instead of being that placid infant with the triple chin of a provincial senator, stuffed in a romper with complicated fastenings, and instead of sleeping away two-thirds of his time in a Moses basket of pale straw with a checked lining, Revol often says to himself that he would have liked to be in the room during the fateful Twenty-Third International Neurology Meeting – the day when Maurice Goulon and Pierre Mollaret climbed into the gallery to share their work. He would have paid good money to see them addressing the medical community; in other words, to see them standing face-to-face with the world itself, these two men, the neurologist and the infectious diseases specialist, forty- and sixty-some years old, dark suits and polished black shoes, bow ties most likely; he would have loved to observe what showed of their relationship, the mutual respect shaded by an age difference that would instate that silent hierarchy common in scientific assemblies, my dear colleague, my dear colleague – but who would speak first? who would have the privilege of concluding? yes, the more Revol thinks about it, the more he would have liked to be there on that day, to take his seat among the pioneers of intensive care, men, mostly, keyed up and concentrating, to be one of them, there, at Claude-Bernard Hospital – a trailblazing hospital: in 1954 Pierre Mollaret would inaugurate the first modern intensive care unit in the world, he would form a team, transform the Pasteur wing to hold nearly seventy beds, would install the famous Engström 150, electric ventilators developed to combat the epidemics of poliomyelitis besieging northern Europe – these would replace the "iron lungs" that had been used since the 1930s; and the more Revol concentrates, the more he fleshes out the scene, this primitive scene that he never witnessed, the better he's able to hear the two professors quietly exchange a few words, arrange their papers on the desk, and clear their throats in front of the microphones; they wait, impassive, for the hubbub to die down, for silence to fall, before finally beginning their talk with that cold clarity of those who, conscious of the fundamental import of what they have to say, abstain from any embellishment and simply describe, describe, describe, playing their conclusions like the ace in poker; and every time he does so, the enormity of their pronouncement stuns him again, explodes in his face. Because what Goulon and Mollaret came to say can be summed up in one sentence, in the form of a slow cluster bomb: the heart stopping is no longer the sign of death, from now on it's the cessation of brain function that is the indication. In other words: if I don't think any-more therefore I am no more. Deposition of the heart and coronation of the brain – a symbolic *coup d'état*, a revolution.

And so the two men addressed the assembly, described the estab-lished signs of what they now call an irreversible coma, detailed several cases of patients whose cardiac and respiratory functions were maintained mechanically by ventilators, even though all brain activity had ceased – patients who, had the resuscitation equipment and techniques for keeping blood flowing to the brain not been per-fected, would have indeed tipped over into cardiac death. They posited that the increase in medical resuscitation had changed the game, that the progress within the discipline required a new defini-tion of death, and they believed that this scientific event – of an incredible philosophical impact – could also pave the way for organ recovery and transplantation.

Goulon and Mollaret's announcement was followed by the publi-cation of a crucial article, in the *Revue neurologique*, that exposed twenty-three cases of irreversible comas – and everyone will remem-ber the titles of those few books in Revol's office, including that review from 1959, it's easy to guess which issue: a document that Revol would have tracked on eBay, bought without bidding, and picked up one November evening at the Lozère-École polytechnique station on the R.E.R. B line – he had paced in the cold for a long time, keeping watch for his seller who finally emerged in the form of a little woman crowned with a topaz turban who scampered along the platform until she reached him, then pocketed the cash, pulled the journal out of a plaid shopping bag, and did her scheming best to swindle him.

*

Riveted once more to his computer screen, Revol takes note of what appears closes his lids, opens them again, and suddenly stands up as though he's about to take off on an approach run. It's 11.40 a.m. when he calls the department front desk, Cordelia Owl picks up, Revol asks her if Simon Limbeau's family has been notified, and the young woman answers yes, the police phoned his mother, she's on her way.

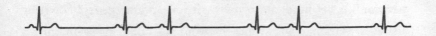

MARIANNE LIMBEAU ENTERS THE HOSPITAL THROUGH THE MAIN doors and walks straight toward the information desk, two women are there seated behind computer screens, two women in light-green shirts who speak quietly to one another. One of them has a thick black braid over her shoulder, she lifts her head to Marianne: hello! Marianne doesn't immediately respond, doesn't know which department to go to – emergency, intensive care, trauma surgery, neurobiology – and struggles to decipher the list of services displayed on a large sign attached to the wall, as though the letters, the words, the lines were overlapping and she couldn't put them back in order, couldn't make sense of them; she finally says: Simon Limbeau. Pardon? The woman frowns – eyebrows thick and also black, they come together in a fuzzy cluster above her nose – Marianne starts again, manages to form a sentence: I'm looking for Simon Limbeau, my son. Ah. On the other side of the counter, the woman leans over the computer and the tip of her braid grazes the keyboard like a Chinese paintbrush: what's the name? Limbeau, L–I–M–B–E–A–U, Marianne spells out and then turns toward the hall, immense, the height of a cathedral and the floor of a skating rink – the acoustics, the sheen, and the marks – scattered pillars, it's quiet here, not many people, a guy in a gown and shower shoes walks with a crutch toward a payphone, a woman in a chair is wheeled around by a man wearing a fedora with an orange feather – a neurasthenic Robin Hood – and far off, near the cafeteria, in front of the row of doors in the dimness, three women in white stand together, plastic cups in hand, I don't see him, when was he admitted? The woman keeps her eyes on the screen and clicks her mouse, this morning, Marianne exhales her answer, the woman lifts her head, oh so maybe it was an emergency? Lowering her eyes, Marianne nods while the woman straightens again, throws her braid over her shoulder and with a wave of her hand indicates the lifts at the end of the hall and the path to follow to get to the emergency department without having to go outside into the cold and all the way around the buildings. Marianne thanks her and continues on her way.

She had fallen back to sleep when the telephone rang, nestled in an interlacing of pale dreams that sifted the light of day and the stridence of synthetic voices from a Japanese animation on the television – later, she would look for signs, in vain: the more she tried to round up the memory, the more her dreams dissolved; she couldn't grasp anything tangible, nothing that could make sense of this shock that happened thirty kilometres away, at the same moment, in the mud of the road – and it wasn't she who answered, it was Lou, seven years old, who came running into her room, not wanting to miss a single moment of the show she was watching in the living room, and who simply put the phone against her mother's ear and then rushed right out again, so that the voice in the receiver wove itself into Marianne's dreams, grew louder, insistent, and it was only when she finally heard these words, please, can you answer me: are you Simon Limbeau's mother? that Marianne sat straight up in bed, brain blinking awake in terror.

She must have screamed loudly, loud enough in any case that the little one reappears, slow and serious, eyes wide, and freezes in the bedroom doorway, head pressed to the doorframe, eyes fixed on her mother who doesn't see her, who pants, like a dog, movements quick and face twisted, tapping furiously on her phone to call Sean who doesn't answer – pick up, pick up, goddammit! – her mother who throws clothes on in a rush, warm boots, huge coat, scarf, then rushes into the bathroom to splash cold water on her face, but no cream, nothing, and when, lifting her head from the sink, she catches her own eye in the mirror – glazed irises beneath lids that are swollen as though by a blow, Simone Signoret eyes, Charlotte Rampling eyes, green line beneath her lashes – and she's struck by not recognising herself, as though her disfiguration had begun, as though she were already a different woman: an entire slice of her life, a massive slice, still warm, compact, detaches from the present and capsizes into the past, plummets and disappears. She makes out piles of rubble, landslides, faults that sever the ground beneath her feet: something is closing off, from now on something is out of reach – a portion of cliff separates from the plateau and crumbles into the sea, a peninsula slowly tears itself from the continent and drifts out to the open, solitary, the door to a magnificent cavern is suddenly obstructed by a rock; the past has grown massive all at once, a life-guzzling ogre, and the present is nothing but an ultra-thin threshold, a line beyond which there is nothing recognisable. The ringing of the phone has cleaved the continuity of time, and before the mirror where her reflection freezes, hands clutching the edges of the sink,

Marianne turns to stone beneath the shock.

Grabbing her purse, she turns around and there is the little girl, she hasn't moved, oh Lou, the child lets herself be hugged without understanding anything, but everything in her is asking her mother questions that she evades, put on your slippers, get a sweater, come with me, and as she slams the apartment door behind them, Marianne suddenly thinks – an icy slash – that the next time she puts her key in the lock, she'll know exactly what's wrong with Simon. On the next floor down, she rings the bell of an apartment, once and then again – Sunday morning, still asleep – and when the woman opens the door, Marianne murmurs hospital, accident, Simon, it's serious, and the woman, eyes widening, nods her head, whispers gently we'll take care of Lou, and the little girl in her pyjamas goes into the apartment, gives a little wave to her mother through the half-open door, but then suddenly changes her mind, throws herself into the stairwell calling: Mama! And Marianne runs back up the stairs, kneels down to face her daughter, takes her in her arms, and then looks deep into her eyes and repeats the cold litany, Simon, surfing, accident, I'll be back, I'll be back soon, the child doesn't blink, places a kiss on her mother's forehead, and goes back into the neighbour's apartment.

Then there is the matter of getting the car out of its spot, second level down in the underground parking lot, and in her panic, it takes two tries to extract herself from the spot, manoeuvering within a millimetre up to the ramp that came out on to the road. The roll-up door opens and she blinks her eyes, blinded. The light of day is white, sallow, it dilutes the dullness, the shitty white of a snowy sky that isn't snowing, and, summoning all her strength and reason, she concentrates on what route to take, driving straight east across the upper part of the city, following arteries as straight-lined as I.V.s penetrating space horizontally, plunging on to rue Félix-Faure, then rue du

329e, then rue Salvador-Allende, names in succession on the route toward the suburbs of Le Havre, names woven into the book that is the city – she passes affluent villas overlooking the cesspool of downtown, vast and perfectly aerated lawns, private institutions and dark sedans, all of this shifting to decrepit buildings, to little suburban houses embellished with verandas or tiny gardens, small paved courtyards where rainwater, mopeds and cases of beer stagnate, and now delivery vans and custom cars glide past these pavements too narrow for two people to pass side by side; she drives past the Tourlaville fort, the funeral parlours beside the cemetery, marble headstones on display behind tall windows, catches sight of a well-lit bakery near Graville Street, a church with open doors – she makes the sign of the cross.

The city was inert, but Marianne could feel the threat – the apprehension of the sailor before a calm sea. It even seemed to her that the space around her had bowed in slightly, in order to contain the phenomenal energy crouching inside matter, this power that could change into a sudden destructive force if anyone came to split open the atoms; but the strangest thing (she had this thought when she looked back later) is that she didn't pass anyone that morning, no other car, no other human being, and not a single animal – dog, cat, rat, insect – the world was deserted, the city emptied of people as though the residents had taken refuge inside their houses to protect themselves from a disaster, as though the war had been lost and they were standing huddled behind their windows to watch the enemy troops pass by, as though each one had quickly moved out of the way of a contagious fatality – anguish pushes people away, everyone knows it – the iron curtain had fallen before the front windows, shades lowered, only the gulls that slackened over the estuary greeted Marianne on her way, whirling above her car that, seen from the sky, was the only moving entity in the whole landscape, mobile capsule that seemed to gather up the last bit of life remaining on earth, shooting out along the ground like the steel ball inside a pinball machine – irreducible, solitary, shaken by spasms. The outside universe dilated slowly, trembled even and paled as the air trembles and pales above the desert sand, above the pavement of roads heated in the sun, it changed into a fleeting, far-off scenery, it whitened, nearly to the point of erasure, while inside the car Marianne drove with one hand, the other wiping away everything that flowed down her face, these tears, stared ahead at the road, tried desperately to ward off the intuition that had been sedimenting in her since the phone call, this intuition that shamed her, that hurt her, and then it was the descent toward Harfleur, the outskirts of Le Havre, the express interchanges where she redoubled her attention, and a closed, unmoving forest – the hospital.

She turned off the car in the parking lot and tried to phone again. Tense, she listened to the regular ring of the call and visualised its pathway: the sound scurried off toward the south of the city, conveyed by a radio wave formed of the invisible air, it crossed the space from one relay mast to the next riding a hertzian frequency that was always different from one to the next, reaching the port and a perimeter of industrial wasteland near the inner harbour, snaked along buildings in disrepair to finally reach that freezing workshop that Marianne didn't visit anymore, not for a long time; she tracked the call that rushed between the palettes and the wood beams, between the chipboard and the plywood panels, mixed with the sound of the wind stuffing itself in through cracked tiles, mixed with the whirlwinds of sawdust and grit spinning in the corners, meddled with the wafts of polyurethane glue, resin or marine varnish, pierced the fibre of heaped-up work shirts and thick leather work gloves, kicked in the tin cans turned paintbrush holders, turned ashtrays, turned kitchen drawers – a fun fair knock 'em down – fought against the continuous vibrations of the circular saw, those of the song on the old ghetto blaster – Rihanna, "Stay" – and against everything that pulsated, twitched, whistled, including the man who worked there, Sean, leaning at this moment over a table with an aluminum rail and evenly spaced abutments to cut boards the same size, a supple, massive man, with weathered hands, who moved slowly, leaving footprints on the powdery ground; equipped with a mask and crowned with an anti-noise helmet, he whistled, like a painter whistles on his ladder, a high melody that curled in the air like the gift ribbon under the scissor blade; she listened to the call that reached the inside pocket of a parka hanging there and released a ring in a telephone casing – the sound of the rain on the surface of the water, a sound he'd downloaded the week before, and that he wouldn't be able to hear.

The ringing stopped, then it was the voicemail box preceded by a horrible jingle. She closed her eyes, the workshop appeared, and suddenly, laid out on metal racks lining the walls, splendid and bronze, the taonga stood out, Sean's treasures: skiffs from the Seine Valley, the umiak, sealskin kayak built by the Inupiat people from northwestern Alaska, and all the wooden canoes that he built there – the largest of them had a finely carved stern like those of the waka, Maori dugouts propelled by long poles and used during ritual processions; the smallest was supple and light, a hull of birch bark and an inside papered with strips of pale wood, Moses' cradle when he was placed upon the Nile to save his life, a nest. It's Marianne, call me back as soon as you can.

Marianne sets off through the lobby. It's long, this crossing, interminable, each step weighted with urgency and fear, she finally reaches the too-large lift, takes it down to the basement, wide corridor, ground lined with wide white tiles, she doesn't pass anyone but can hear women's voices speaking to each other, the hallway turns and reveals a crowd of people who come and go, standing, sitting, lying in wheeled beds parked against the walls, diffuse activity where complaints and murmurs weave together, the voice of a man who's growing impatient, I've been waiting over an hour, the trembling of an old woman veiled in black, the cries of a child in the arms of its mother.

A door is open, it's a windowed office. Again a young woman sitting in front of a computer who lifts a round face toward her, a very open face, maybe twenty-five years old, no more, it's a nurse intern, Marianne says I'm Simon Limbeau's mother, the young woman frowns, disconcerted, then pivots on her chair to speak to someone behind her: Simon Limbeau, a young man, admitted this morning, know where he is? The man turns around, shakes his head no, and seeing Marianne says to the nurse: try calling the I.C.U. The young woman picks up the receiver, enquires, hangs up again, nods, and then the man comes out of the office, a movement that releases a shot of adrenalin somewhere in Marianne's belly, she suddenly feels hot, unties her scarf and opens her coat, wipes away the sweat pearled on her forehead, it's suffocating in here, the man holds out a hand, he's small and frail, neck of a fledgling in a pale-pink shirt with a collar that's too big, his white coat clean and buttoned, the badge with his name placed neatly on his chest. Marianne holds out her hand too, but can't help wondering if it's just custom or if this movement, however banal, manifests an intention, a solicitude or something else, motivated by Simon's state, when she doesn't actually want to hear anything, know anything, not yet, doesn't want to listen to any information that would come to alter the affirmation "your son is alive".

The doctor pulls her down the corridor toward the lifts, Marianne bites her lip while he continues: he's not in this department, he was admitted straightaway to intensive care – his nasal voice crushes "a"s and "en"s, his tone is neutral, Marianne stops, eyes staring, voice breaking: he's in intensive care? Yes. The doctor moves soundlessly, taking small steps in crepe-soled shoes, he floats inside his white coat, his waxy nose gleams in the light, and Marianne, who is a head taller than him, makes out the skin of his scalp beneath thin hair. He crosses his hands behind his back: I can't tell you anything more, but come along, they'll explain everything, no doubt he was admitted there because of the state he was in. Marianne closes her eyes and grits her teeth, suddenly everything within her retracts, if she keeps speaking she'll scream, or else throw herself at him and smack her hand over his stupidly verbose mouth, please God let him shut up, and as though by magic he lets his sentence trail off, wordless, and stops in front of her, head wobbling on the collar of the pink shirt; stiff as cardboard, his hand comes up palm open toward the ceiling – a vague gesture in which all the contingency of the world fans out, the fragility of human existence – then falls back beside his leg: the I.C.U. knows you're on your way, someone will come to meet you. They've reached the lifts and the meeting comes to an end; the doctor indicates the other end of the corridor with a movement of his chin, and concludes, calm but firm, I have to go, it's Sunday, emergency is always crowded on Sundays, people don't know quite what to do, he presses the button, the metal doors open slowly, and suddenly, while their hands are once again shaking each other, he smiles at Marianne, a smile from rock bottom, goodbye ma'am, be brave, and turns back toward the cries.

*

43

He said be brave, Marianne repeats these words to herself while she goes up another floor – the path to Simon is long, these hospitals like labyrinths are trying – the lift is papered with signs and union flyers, be brave, he said be brave, her eyelids stick together, her hands are damp, and the pores of her skin open because of the heat, a cutaneous dilation that disturbs her features, goddamn "be brave", goddamn heat, isn't there any air to breathe?

The intensive care unit takes up the whole east wing of the main floor. Access is restricted, signs saying Hospital Personnel Only are posted on doors, so Marianne waits in the corridor, ends up leaning against the wall and letting herself slide down to a crouch, head moving right and left without lifting from the wall, she taps her head against it, digs in gently with her occiput, face lifted toward the fluorescent tubes that run along the ceiling, lids closed, she listens, always these busy voices that jibe or update each other from one end of the corridor to the other, these feet in rubber soles, gymnastics shoes, or ordinary little sneakers, these metallic jinglings, these ringing alarms, these rolling stretchers, the continuous rustle of the place. She checks her phone: Sean hasn't called. She decides to move, she has to go, approaches the double fire door edged in black rubber, stands on tiptoe to look through the window. It's quiet. She opens the door and goes inside.

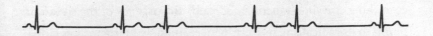

HE KNEW RIGHT AWAY WHO SHE WAS — STUNNED LOOK, EYES IN
in a tailspin, cheeks bitten from inside — so he didn't ask if she
was Simon Limbeau's mother, just held out his hand and nodded
his head: Pierre Revol, I'm a doctor in the department, I'm the one
who admitted your son this morning, come with me. She walks with
her head turned instinctively down toward the linoleum, without a
glance to either side that might slip off to find her child at the back of
some dark room, twenty metres to the end of the pale-blue corridor
and then an ordinary door with a label in the form of a visitor's card,
and written on it, a name she can't make out.

This Sunday, Revol spurns the family room, which he doesn't
much like, and instead invites Marianne into his office. She stays
standing, finally sits on the edge of the chair as he walks around the
desk to slide into his seat, chest forward, elbows spread. The more
Marianne observes him, the more the other faces she's seen since her
arrival disappear, the woman with the unibrow at the front desk, the
young nurse intern in emergency, the doctor with the pink collar — as
though they had only spelled each other off until they led her to this
face, superimposed one on top of the other until they formed only a
single one, the face of the man sitting in front of her, ready to speak.

*

Would you like a coffee? Marianne jumps, nods. Revol gets up, and turning his back to her picks up the coffee pot that she hadn't seen, pours the coffee into white Styrofoam cups, it steams, his movements are wide and silent, sugar? He's buying time, arranging his words, she knows this, and goes along with the tempo, feels the paradoxical tension as time drips out like coffee from the coffee-maker while everything else simultaneously screams the urgency of the situation, points to its radicalism, its imminence, and now Marianne has closed her eyes, she drinks, concentrating on the liquid burning her throat, this is how much she dreads the first word of the first sentence – the jaw moving, the lips that open and stretch, the teeth that show, sometimes the tip of the tongue – this sentence saturated with sorrow that she knows is about to be formed, everything in her recoils and defects, her spine presses against the back of the chair – wobbly – her head leans back, she wishes she could get out of here, run to the door and escape, or disappear into a trap-door that might suddenly open beneath the legs of her chair, poof! a hole, an oubliette – wishes she could be forgotten herself, yes, and that no one would be able to find her and that she'd never know anything other than Simon's beating heart – she wishes she could leave this cramped room, this dismal light, and run from the announcement, she's not brave, no, she writhes inside and zigzags like a grass snake, she would give anything to have someone just reassure her, just lie to her, tell her a story with some suspense, sure, but with an acidulous happy ending, she's shamefully cowardly, but holds firm: every second that passes is another bit of war spoils, every second that goes by stops destiny in its tracks, and as he sees these agitated hands, these legs knotted beneath the chair, these closed swollen lids, smudged with yesterday's makeup – a coal-grey eyeshadow that she applies to her lids with the tip of her finger, with a single gesture – the blurred transparency of these irises is touching, a cloudy aquatic jade, and the trembling of her splayed lashes, Revol knows that she understands, knows that she knows, and it's with infinite gentleness that he consents to stretch out the time that precedes his words, picking up the Venetian paperweight and rolling it in his palm: the ball of glass sparkles under the cold fluorescent light, rainbows the walls and ceiling, venous, it passes over Marianne's face and she opens her eyes, and that is Revol's sign that he can begin.

– Your son's condition is serious.

At the first words uttered – clear timbre, calm cadence – Marianne presses her eyes – dry – into Revol's own and he looks back at her, steady, even as his phrase sets to swaying, even as it's composed, crystal-clear without being brutal – semantics of a direct precision, *largo* woven in with silences, a slowing that weds itself to the unfolding of meaning – slow enough that Marianne can repeat each of the syllables inwardly, inscribe them in herself: during the accident, your son suffered a head injury, the scanner shows a serious lesion on the frontal lobe – he brings his hand to his head, at the top of his forehead, illustrating his words – and this trauma caused a cerebral haemorrhage – Simon was in a coma when he arrived at the hospital.

The coffee cools in the cup, Revol drinks slowly and, before him, Marianne has become a stone statue. The telephone reverberates in the room, one, two, three rings, but Revol doesn't answer, Marianne stares at his face, absorbs every detail – silky white complexion, mauve circles below large transparent grey saucers, heavy eyelids creased like nutshells, a long and turbulent face – and the silence swells, until Revol begins again: I'm worried – his voice surprises her, inexplicably loud, as though its volume had malfunctioned – we're doing tests at the moment, and the first results are not good – although his voice makes an unfamiliar sound in Marianne's ear and instantly causes her breathing to accelerate, it's not cloying, doesn't sound like those disgusting voices that pretend to comfort while they're pushing you into the charnel house, instead it marks out a place for Marianne, a place and a line.

– He's in a deep coma.

The seconds that follow open up a space between them, a naked and silent space, and they stay at the edge for a long moment. Marianne Limbeau begins slowly to turn the word "coma" over in her mind while Revol returns to the bleak part of his work; the millefiori still rolls in his palm, smoky and solitary sun, and nothing has ever seemed more violent, more complex than coming to sit beside this woman so they can delve together into this fragile zone of language where death announces itself, so they can go forward into it, together. He says: Simon is not responding to painful stimuli anymore, he's demonstrating abnormal ocular and vegetative symptoms, and in particular an abnormal breathing pattern, with early signs of pulmonary congestion, and the initial brain scans are not good – his sentence is slow, punctuated with pauses for breath, a way of situating his body in the moment, making it present in his speech, a way of turning a clinical statement into an instance of empathy; he speaks as though he were carving some material, and now they hold each other's gaze, face each other, that's it, that's exactly what this is, an absolute face-off, unflinching, as though speaking and looking at each other were two sides of the same coin, as though it were a matter of facing each other as much as facing that which was happening in one of these hospital rooms.

I want to see Simon – panicked, the voice, the eyes out of control, hands that scatter. I want to see Simon, that's all she said, while her phone vibrated for the umpteenth time in the bottom of her coat pocket – the neighbour who's taking care of Lou, Chris's parents, Johan's, but still no word from Sean, where is he? She types out a text: call me.

Revol has lifted his head: now, you want to see him now? He casts a quick look at his watch – 12.30 – and answers, calmly, you can't see him right now, it will be a short wait, he's undergoing a procedure, but as soon as we're finished, of course you can see your son. And placing a yellowed piece of paper in front of him, he continues: if you don't mind, I need to talk to you a little bit about Simon. Talk about Simon. Marianne grows tense. What does he mean, "talk about Simon?" Does it mean giving information about his body like you'd give information on an application? Marking out the operations he's had – adenoids, appendicitis, that's it; the fractures? A broken radius falling off his bike the summer he was ten, that's all; allergies that affect his daily life? No, none; infections he's contracted? Golden staph in the summer he was five, which he announced to everyone, enshrouded with the glow of rarity this spectacular name granted him, mononucleosis at sixteen, the kissing disease, the lovers' disease, and he smiled slantways when people teased him, all that month he wore some strange pyjamas, a combination of Hawaiian shorts and a quilted sweatshirt. Does it mean listing off childhood diseases? Talk about Simon. Images wash over her, Marianne panics: the rose-ola of a baby in a garter-stitch-knit sweater, the chicken pox of a three-year-old, brown crusty scabs on his scalp, behind his ears, that fever that had dehydrated him and left the whites of his eyes yellow and his hair sticky for ten days. Marianne utters monosyllables while Revol takes a few notes – date and place of birth, weight, height – and he seems not to care too much about childhood diseases once he's noted that Simon has no particular medical history, no serious illnesses, rare allergies, or malformations that his mother knows of – at these words Marianne grows agitated, a flash of memory, a ski outing with his class to the Contamines-Montjoie, Simon was ten and had a terrible pain in his abdomen, the doctor at the ski hill who examined him palpated his left side and, suspecting appendicitis, diagnosed an "inversed anatomy", in other words the heart on the right side and everything else in keeping, words that no one had ever doubted, and this fantastic anomaly had given him extraspecial status right through to the end of the trip.

Thank you; then, having smoothed the paper with the flat of his hand, he places it back inside Simon's file, a pale-green folder. He lifts his head toward Marianne, you can see your son as soon as we've finished the tests. What tests? Marianne's voice straight ahead in the office and the vague idea that if they are doing tests then nothing is sure yet. The radiance of her gaze alerts Revol, who forces himself to keep the situation in check and to curb hope: Simon's state is progressive, and this progression is not headed in the right direction. Marianne is knocked off course, says oh, so what is Simon's state progressing toward? As she says it, she knows she's revealing her vulnerability, she's taking a risk, and Revol takes a breath before replying.

– Simon's lesions are irreversible.

Revol has the painful feeling of dealing a blow, the sense of detonating a bomb. And then he gets up, we'll call you as soon as possible, and adds, a little more loudly, has Simon's father been informed?

Marianne hooks him with her eyes, he'll be here around noon, but Sean doesn't call, still no word, and Marianne is suddenly seized by panic, tells herself maybe he's not at the workshop, maybe he's not even at home, maybe he left to deliver a skiff in Villequier, Duclair, or Caudebec-en-Caux, or to a rowing club on the Seine, and maybe at this exact moment he was aboard the vessel, demonstrating it to a buyer, and they were rowing, sitting on swivel seats, observing how it handled and commenting on it in low tones, using an expert's vocabulary, and little by little Marianne sees the river's course narrowing between high rock walls suckered by thick mosses, masses of plants growing horizontally, giant ferns and thick creepers, sphagnum moss, plants of a brilliant green tangled together along vertiginous walls or bowing toward the river in vegetal cascades, and then it grows dim, the cliffs leaving only a thin corridor of sky white as milk, the water grows heavy, flat and slow, surface saturated with insects – dragonflies iridescent with turquoise, transparent mosquitoes – it turns bronze, dull with silver flashes, and suddenly, horrified, Marianne imagines that Sean has gone back to New Zealand, and that he is headed up the Whanganui River from Cook Strait, setting off from another estuary and another city, and that he is heading deeper into the interior, alone in his canoe, absolutely peaceful, peaceful as she had known him to be, serene eyes; his movements regular, he passes Maori villages along the banks, portages around waterfalls, the light craft hoisted on his back, and advances farther and farther to the north, toward the central plateau and the Tongariro Volcano, where the sacred river drew its source, retracing the path of the migration to new lands; she sees Sean clearly, and even hears his breath swell in the canyon as in an echo chamber, where reigns a suffocating calm – Revol watches her, worried by her panicked face, but needing to wrap up, so I'll see you with him then, and Marianne nods her head, okay.

Scrape of chairs against the floor, creak of the door hinges, they walk toward the end of the corridor, and once they're in the doorway, without adding a sentence to their meagre dialogue, Marianne pivots and moves away slowly without knowing where to go, passes the waiting room, straight chairs and a low table cluttered with well-thumbed magazines, mature women smiling from the covers with healthy teeth, shining hair, toned perineums, and soon here she is under the immense nave of glass and concrete once again, on the tiles with thousands of scuff marks, she passes the cafeteria – multi-coloured bags of crisps, sweets and chewing gum on display shelves, pizzas and burgers in primary colours on signs aligned neatly above, bottles of water and pop standing in windowed fridges – stops suddenly, sways on her feet, Simon is lying in there somewhere, how can she leave him behind? She wants to turn back, but she keeps going, she needs to find Sean, she has to reach him at all costs.

She heads for the main door that opens slowly, far off; four figures cross the threshold and come toward her, figures that soon emerge from the blur cast by her myopic eyes: it's the parents of the other two *caballeros*, Christophe and Johan, the four of them in a line, and again the winter coats that weigh shoulders down, the scarves rolled into neck braces to hold up falling heads, the gloves. They recognise her, slow down, and then one of the men quickens his step to break rank and when he reaches Marianne folds her in his arms, and then the other three hug her in turn. How is he? Chris's father is the first to speak; the four of them look at her, she's paralysed. Murmurs: he's in a coma, we don't know yet. She shrugs her shoulders and her mouth distorts: and you? the boys? Johan's mother answers: Chris, fractured left hip and fibula; Johan, both wrists and clavicle fractured, also his ribcage, but none of his organs were pierced – she remains sober, of an outrageous sobriety, meant to show Marianne that the four of them are aware of how lucky they are, of their monster's ball, because for them, it's only breakage – their children were wearing seat belts, were protected from the shock, and if this woman minimises their anxiety to this extent, abstaining from any commentary, it's also to show Marianne that they know about Simon, know that it's serious, very serious even, a rumour that will have run from the I.C.U. to the department of orthopaedic and trauma surgery where their sons are, and that she won't have the indecency to add anything, and finally, there is this distress she feels, this guilt that holds her back, because the choice was between their two sons, for the seat belt – Chris had to drive, so it could just as easily have been Johan in the middle and then she would be the one in Marianne's place at this instant, exactly in her place, swaying before the same terrible abyss, disfigured in just the same way, and she's suddenly dizzy at the thought, her legs go weak and her eyes begin to roll back, and her husband moves closer, feeling her wavering, puts an arm under hers to steady her, and as Marianne sees this woman capsize, she, too, perceives the abyss between them, between herself and the rest of them, this chasm that separates them now, thank you, I have to go, we'll keep you posted.

She suddenly realises that she doesn't want to go home, it's not time yet to see Lou, to call her mother, to tell Simon's grandparents, his friends, it's not time to hear them panic and suffer, some of them will scream into the receiver, no, oh my god, oh shit, goddammit I can't believe it, some of them will burst into sobs while others will barrage her with questions, say the names of medical tests she won't know, tell her about the case of an acquaintance who woke up from a coma when they thought he was lost, and they'll round up all the spectacular remissions in their circle and beyond, will be suspicious of the hospital, the diagnosis and the treatment, and will even ask the name of the doctor who received him, ah, well, I don't recognise that name, oh him, I don't know him, oh he's probably very good, and will insist that she write down the number of that amazing hospital practitioner who has a two-year wait-list, may even offer to call him themselves, since they know him or have a friend who, and maybe there will even be someone stupid enough – someone completely out to lunch – to tell her that it's possible, it happens, to get an irreversible coma mixed up with other states that resemble it – the alcoholic coma, for example, an overdose of sedatives, hypoglycaemia, or even hypothermia – and then, remembering the surf session in cold water that very morning, she'll feel like vomiting but will get hold of herself to remind the person tormenting her that there was an extremely violent accident, and although she will resist, repeating to everyone that Simon is in good hands, that we just have to wait, they'll still want to shower her with affection and cover her with words, no, it's not that time yet, what she wants is some place to wait, a place to exhaust time, she wants some shelter, reaches the parking lot and suddenly begins to run toward her car, dives inside, and then it's fists pounding against the steering wheel and her hair that flies over the dashboard, actions that are so disordered she has trouble putting the key in the ignition, and when she finally starts the car, she jolts forward, screeches her tyres in the parking lot, then drives straight out, toward the west, toward the west wind, the sky keeps getting clearer over this city, while back in his office Revol doesn't sit down but does what the law requires him to do when an encephalic death is announced in I.C.U.: he picks up his phone, composes the number for the organ and tissue donation programme, and it's Thomas Remige who picks up.

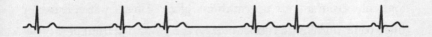

BUT HE ALMOST MISSED THE CALL, HE NEARLY DIDN'T HEAR IT, and it was during a pause to catch his breath at the end of a long lively phrase – a vocal polyphony, a flight of birds, Benjamin Britten, *A Ceremony of Carols*, Op. 28 – that he caught the chirp-chirp of the phone that was echoed, brilliantly and delicately, by a goldfinch in its cage.

That Sunday morning, in a garden studio on rue Commandant-Charcot, Thomas Remige makes the slats of a venetian blind quiver; he is alone, naked, and he's singing. He stands in the centre of the room – always in the same spot – his body weight spread equally over both feet, back straight, shoulders held lightly back, ribcage open to free the chest and neck; once he's steady, makes a few slow circular movements with his head to loosen his cervical spine, repeats these same rotations with each shoulder, then begins to visualise the column of air that armatures him, from the pit of his belly to his throat, this internal conduit that powers the breath and will make his vocal cords vibrate; he refines his posture. Finally he opens his mouth, an oven – a little odd at the moment, vaguely ridiculous – fills his lungs with air, contracts his abdominal wall, then exhales, an action like opening a gate, and stretches this action out as long as possible, mobilising his diaphragm and his zygomatics – a deaf person would have been able to listen simply by placing their hands on him. If you were there to witness the scene, you might see a link with the sun salutation or the morning ritual of monks and nuns, this lyricism of the dawn; you might see any corporal ritual intended to maintain and conserve the body – drinking a glass of fresh water, brushing one's teeth, unrolling a rubber mat on the ground in front of the tele- vision to do some stretches – but for Thomas Remige, this is something completely different: it is an exploration of the self – his voice like a probe inserted in the body and causing everything that animates him to reverberate on the surface, his voice like a stetho- scope.

He was twenty when he left the family farm, a well-to-do plot in Nor- mandy that his sister and brother-in-law would eventually take over. Bye-bye school bus and mud in the yard, smell of wet hay, the solitary moo of a cow demanding to be milked and the border of poplars grown close together on a grassy bank, from now on he lives in a tiny studio that his parents rent to him in downtown Rouen, electric radi- ator and pull-out couch, rides a Honda 500 from 1971, has started nursing school, likes girls, likes boys, doesn't know, and one night during a jaunt to Paris goes to a karaoke bar in Belleville, there are several Chinese people there, vinyl hair and waxy cheeks, regulars come to polish their performances, couples, mostly, who admire and film each other, re-enacting dance moves and postures from T.V. shows, and suddenly, succumbing to the pressure of his friends, here he is choosing a song, a short thing, a simple thing – I think it was "It's a Heartache" by Bonnie Tyler – and when his turn comes he goes onstage, and slowly metamorphoses: little by little, his abulic body settles, a voice comes out of his mouth, a voice that's his but one he doesn't recognise, incredible timbre, texture and range, as though his body housed other versions of himself – a wild cat, a jagged cliff, a lady of the night – and the DJ isn't mistaken, it really is him singing, and then, taking hold of his voice as his body signature, taking hold of his voice as the shape of his singularity, he decides to get to know himself and begins to sing.

Discovering singing, he discovers his body, that's how it happens. Like the sports amateur after an intense session – running, cycling, gymnastics – he feels tightnesses he hasn't felt before, knots and currents, points and zones, as though something of himself is being revealed – his unexplored potential. He endeavours to recognise everything that composes him, conceiving of the precise anatomy, the shape of the organs, the variety of muscles, their unsuspected resources; he explores his respiratory system, and how the action of singing pulls him together and holds him, raises him up into a human body and perhaps even more, into a singing body. It's a rebirth.

The time and money he consecrates to singing swells over the course of years, coming to take up a consequential part of his daily life and a salary beefed up by extra shifts at the hospital: he vocalises every morning, studies every night, takes a class twice a week with an opera singer who has a body shaped like a light bulb – giraffe neck and reed-thin arms, strapping pelvis and flat belly, chest in proportion, voluminous, all of this sheltered beneath hair that undulates down to her knees, hurtling down flannel skirts – at night tracks this or that recital, opera, new recording, downloads everything, pirates, copies, archives, in the summer crosses France to go here and there, an opera festival, sleeps in a tent or shares a rented bungalow with other enthusiasts like him, meets Ousmane, a Gnawa musician with a shimmering baritone voice, and suddenly last summer it was a trip to Algeria and the acquisition of a goldfinch in the Collo Valley – he drops the whole of his inheritance from his grandmother on these two things – three thousand euros in cash rolled inside a cambric handkerchief.

His first years as an intensive care unit nurse shake his foundations: he enters an otherworldly space, a subterranean or parallel world, at the edge of the other one and disturbed by their adjacency, continuously brushing against one another, this world that's punctuated by a thousand slumbers, but where he never sleeps. In the early days, he criss-crosses the department as you'd explore your own internal cartography, conscious that he's encountering the other half of time, the cerebral night, the heart of things, the reactor core – his voice grows clearer, grows richer in nuance, it was then that he was studying his first *Lied*, a Brahms lullaby, in fact, a simple song that he probably sang for the first time at the bedside of a restless patient, the melody like a tactile analgesic. Flexible hours, heavy responsibilities, shortages of everything: the department is a closed space, with its own set of rules, and Thomas has the feeling of cutting himself off bit by bit from the outside world, of living in a place where the caesura of night and day doesn't affect him anymore. He sometimes feels he's losing ground. To get some air, he multiplies the intensives from which he emerges worn out but ballasted by a deepening gaze and a voice that is ever richer, working hard without ever banking any energy, and he's starting to be noticed in the department meetings, mastering procedures calibrated to the various phases of sleep, including the waking phase, carefully manipulating monitors and life-support devices, taking an interest in pain management. Seven years of this rhythm and then the desire to gravitate in a different direction within this same perimeter. He becomes one of the three hundred organ donation specialists in the country, goes to join the hospital in Le Havre, he's twenty-nine, he's magnificent. When asked about this new direction which required, as one would imagine, supplementary training, Thomas answers: contact with patients' loved ones, psychology, law, the collective aspect, everything that abounds in his career as a nurse, sure, sure, but there's something else, something more complex, and if he feels he's with someone he can trust, if he chooses to take his time, he'll speak of this singular sensation of feeling your way on the threshold of the living, of a questioning about the human body and its uses, of an approach to death and its representations – because that's what this is about. He ignores the friends who badger and jibe – and what if the electroencephalogram was wrong, eh, a malfunction, a momentary crash, an electrical problem, right, and if the guy wasn't really dead, that happens sometimes, right? Whoa, you're messing with death, Tom, that's kinda sketchy, kinda dark – chews the end of his umpteenth matchstick and smiles, buys a round the night he receives, with honours, his master's in philosophy from the Sorbonne – swashbuckling specialist of shift-trading with co-workers, he was able to find someone to fill in for him during those five half-day seminars held in the rue Saint-Jacques, a street he liked to take all the way to the Seine, listening to the rustling of the city, singing sometimes.

Impossible to know what today will bring, Thomas Remige is on standby, the I.C.U. could call at any moment during his twenty-four hours, that's the principle. Like every time, he has to reconcile himself to these hours that are at once vacant but unavailable – these paradoxical hours that are perhaps the other name for boredom – has to organise latency, and often screws it up, managing neither to rest nor take advantage of this free time, suspended in a state of expectancy, paralysed by procrastination – he prepares himself to leave, to finally rest; begins a cake, a film, an archive of digital sounds – the song of the goldfinch – ends up ditching, rewinding, leaving it aside and postponing, we'll see later, but later never exists, later is a flow of full time all stirred up by irregular hours. Also, seeing the hospital's number on the screen of his phone, Thomas feels both a pang of disappointment and a simultaneous sense of relief.

The organ donation unit that he's in charge of functions as an independent department even though it's situated inside the hospital walls, but Revol and Remige know each other, and the young man knows exactly what Revol is about to tell him, he could even utter it for him, this sentence that standardises tragedy for better efficiency: a patient in the unit has been pronounced brain-dead. A statement that sounds like a concluding sentence, when it's not so for Thomas, no, it's a different meaning that it lays out, indicating on the contrary the beginning of series of movements, the launch of a process.

– A patient in the unit has been pronounced brain-dead.

Revol's voice recites the script to a T. Okay, Remige seems to answer, he doesn't open his mouth but nods his head, instantly going over the ultracalibrated process he's about to to set in motion within a legal framework that is both dense and strict, a high-precision movement unfolded along a precise temporal line, and here he is looking at his watch – an action he'll repeat several times in the hours that follow, an action they will all repeat, incessantly, up until the end.

A dialogue ensues, quick, alternating sentences spoken alongside the body of Simon Limbeau, Remige polling Revol on three points: the context of the brain-death diagnosis – where are we with that? – the medical evaluation of the patient – cause of death, medical history, feasibility of organ retrieval – and finally, the family – has it been possible to speak with them yet, given the violence of the event? is the family present? Revol responds to this last question in the negative and then specifies, I just met the mother. Okay, I'll get ready, Remige shivers, he's cold – he is naked, after all – remember?

A few moments later, helmet, gloves and boots on, jacket buttoned up to the neck and his indigo scarf wound round his neck, Thomas Remige mounts his motorcycle, sets off in the direction of the hospital – before donning his helmet, he will have listened to the echo of his steps in the silent street, paying close attention to this impression of a canyon, of a sonorous bottleneck. A flick of his wrist starts his engine, and then he zooms eastward following the straight road that divides this part of the city – a road parallel to the one Marianne took only a little while before him – diving into rue René-Coty, Maréchal-Joffre, Aristide-Briand – names with goatees and moustaches, names with paunches and pocket watches, names with floppy hats – rue Verdun and all the way to the freeway at the edge of the city. His full-face helmet prevents him from singing, and yet, some days, prey to this sort of overflowing based in both fear and euphoria, he goes full-tilting along urban corridors, visor lifted, and uses his vocal cords to make space vibrate.

*

Later, at the hospital, Thomas knows this lobby with its oceanic dimensions by heart, this emptiness that he must cleave in one shot, drawing a diagonal across the space to reach the stairway that leads to his office, the organ and tissue donation programme, on the second floor. But this morning, he enters as a stranger might, as alert as an outsider, he arrives here the way he arrives at other hospitals in the area – establishments without the capacity to do transplants. Speeds up past the counter where two men wait, silent, eyes red, jeans and big black down jackets, lifts a hand in greeting to the woman with the unibrow and she, seeing him show up when she knows he's on call, guesses that a patient in the I.C.U. just became a potential donor, contents herself with just a look in response – the arrival of the organ donation specialist is always a delicate sequence: the patient's loved ones, oblivious to what is unfolding, might overhear her telling someone the reason for his presence, and might link this to the state of their child, their brother, their lover, be blindsided, staggered, which wouldn't bode well for the meetings to come.

Revol stands behind his desk, in his lair, hands Thomas the medical file for Simon Limbeau with a raise of his eyebrows – his eyes grow big, his forehead creases – and speaks to him as though he were picking up their telephone conversation where it left off: nineteen-year-old kid, non-reactive neurological exam, not responsive to pain, cranial nerve reflexes absent, fixed pupils, haemodynamically stable, I've seen the mother, the father will be arriving in about two hours. The specialist casts a glance at his watch, two hours? Again the dregs from the coffeepot splatsplat in a squeaky cup. Revol continues: I just asked for the first E.E.G. (electroencephalogram) it's in process, words that crack like the starter's gun – in ordering this test, Revol shows that he's begun the legal procedure to certify death in the young man. Two types of protocol are at his disposal, either an angiogram by brain scanner or, in the case of a brain death, an X-ray that would confirm the absence of liquid inside the skull, or else two thirty-minute E.E.G.s, done at an interval of four hours, and showing the flat line that illustrates the absence of all brain activity. Thomas picks up the signal and says: we'll be able to proceed to a complete evaluation of the organs. Revol nods his head, I know.

In the corridor, they go their separate ways. Revol heads toward the recovery room to check on the patients admitted that morning, while Remige goes back to his office and immediately opens the green folder. He dives in, turning the pages with great attention – the information given by Marianne, the emergency team's summary, the tests and scans from today – he memorises the numbers and compares the data. Little by little, he forms a clear idea of the state of Simon's body. A kind of apprehension comes over him: although he knows the steps and the milestones of the process he's beginning, he also knows to what extent it differs from a well-oiled mechanism, a chain of set phrases and diagonal checkmarks on a checklist. This is *terra incognita.*

And then he clears his throat and calls the French Agency of Biomedicine in Saint-Denis. We're at that point.

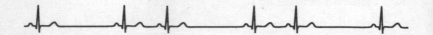

THE STREET TOO IS SILENT, SILENT AND MONOCHROMATIC AS the rest of the world. The catastrophe has spread over the elements, places, things, a curse, as though everything has conformed to what had happened this morning, behind the cliffs – the garish van smashed at full speed against the pole and this kid thrown headfirst against the windshield – as though the outside had absorbed the impact of the accident, had engulfed the aftershocks, muffled the last vibrations, as though the shock wave had stretched out, diminished, weakened until it became a flat line, this single line that raced out into space to mix with all the others, joined the billions and billions of other lines that form the violence of the world, this cluster of sorrows and ruin, and as far as the eye can see, nothing, not a touch of light, not a splash of bright colour, golden yellow, carmine red, not a song slipped from an open car window – a bounding rock song or a melody whose chorus we join in, laughing, happy and a little ashamed to know such sentimental words by heart – no scent of coffee, flowers, or spices, nothing, not a single child with red cheeks running after a ball or crouched chin-to-knees following a marble with his eyes as it rolls along the pavement, not a shout, no human voices calling to each other or murmuring words of love, no cry of a newborn, not a single living being caught up in the continuity of days, occupied with the simple and insignificant acts of a winter morning: nothing comes to insult Marianne's suffering as she moves forward like an automaton, with a mechanical step and a hazy look. On this fateful day. She repeats these words to herself in a low voice, doesn't know where they come from, she says them with her eyes glued to the tips of her boots, as though the words accompanied the muted beat, a regular sound that spares her from having to think beyond this moment, this one task: take one step then another and another then sit down and drink. She heads slowly toward the café she knows is open on Sunday, a shelter she reaches at the limits of her strength. On this fateful day, I pray to you, O my God. She whispers these words in a loop, separating out their syllables like the beads on a rosary, how long has it been since she said a prayer out loud? She wishes she could keep walking forever.

She pushes open the door. It's dark inside, traces of nocturnal drifts, smell of cooled ashes. Alain Bashung sings. *Voleur d'amphores au fond des criques*, (thief of amphorae at the bottom of creeks). She goes to the counter, leans over the zinc, she's thirsty, doesn't want to wait, is anyone here? A guy comes out of the kitchen, enormous, a cotton sweatshirt stretched tight across his belly, loose jeans, dishevelled shock of hair like he just rolled out of bed, yeah, yeah, there's someone here, and once he's in front of her he starts up again formal so, miss, what are we having? A gin – Marianne's voice, barely audible, an exhalation. The guy slicks his hair back with two heavily ringed hands, then rinses a glass all the while slanting a glance at this woman out of the corner of his eye, sure he's seen her here before: everything alright, miss? Marianne turns her eyes away, I'm going to sit down.

The large spotted mirror at the end of the room reflects a face she doesn't recognise, she turns her head away.

Don't close your eyes, listen to the song, count the bottles above the counter, observe the shape of the glasses, puzzle out the posters. *Où subsiste encore ton écho,* (where an echo of you still remains). Create decoys, divert the violence. Build a dam against the images of Simon that form rapidly and crash into her in successive waves, in a great sweep, push them away, beat them back if you can, while already they're organising into memories, nineteen years of memory sequences, a mass. Stave them off. The flashes of memory that arose when she talked about Simon in Revol's cubbyhole had lodged a pain in her chest that she was powerless to control or diminish – for that, she would have had to locate the memory in her brain, inject a paralysing fluid, the needle guided by a high-precision computer – but all she would find there would be the motor of the action, the ability to remember, because memory itself is actually held in the body as a whole, Marianne didn't know this. *J'ai fait la saison dans cette boîte crânienne,* (I spent the whole season inside this cranium). She has to think, gather things together and reorder them so she can utter a clear phrase to Sean when he arrives, spared as yet. Chain the propositions together intelligibly. First: Simon has been in an accident. Second: He's in a coma – gulp of gin. *Dresseur de loulous, dynamiteur d'aqueducs,* (Spitz trainer, dynamiter of aqueducts.) Third: The situation is irreversible – she swallows, thinking about this word she'll have to speak aloud, "irreversible", five syllables that vitrify the state of things and that she never, ever says, believing in the continual movement of life, the possible reversal of every situation, nothing is irreversible, nothing, she has the habit of saying time and time again – and usually she says it lightly, swaying the phrase as you would gently shake someone who was discouraged, nothing is

66

irreversible, except death, disability, and maybe then she would even get up and spin around, maybe she would even dance. But Simon – no. For Simon, it's irreversible.

Sean's face – these tapered eyes beneath heavy lids – lights up on the screen of her phone. Marianne, you called me. Immediately she dissolves into tears – chemistry of grief – incapable of articulating a single word while he says again: Marianne? Marianne? He must have thought that the echo of the sea cramped inside the inner harbour was interfering, he must have confused the drool, snot and tears with static on the radio waves while she bit the back of her hand, paralysed by the horror that suddenly rose in her at the sound of this voice, so dear, familiar as only a voice can be – but suddenly estranged, abominably estranged, because it arises from a space–time where Simon's accident never happened, a world intact, situated light years from this empty café; and it was dissonant now, this voice, it disorchestrated the world, it tore at her brain: it was the voice of life before. Marianne hears this man calling her and she weeps, swept through with the emotion we sometimes feel when faced with that which has survived unscathed, in time – it unleashes the pain of the impossibility of going back. One day she will have to learn which direction time flows, if it's linear or if it traces the rapid circles of a hula hoop, if it forms rings, rolls in upon itself like the whorls of a shell, if it can take the form of the tube that bends the wave, sucks up the sea and the entire universe in its dark backhand, yes, she will have to understand what it's made of, the time that passes. Marianne grips her phone in her hand: scared to speak, scared to destroy Sean's voice, scared that she will never again be allowed to hear it as it is, that she will never again be allowed to experience this disappeared time where Simon was not in an irreversible situation, knowing full well that she has to put an end to the anachronism of this voice and reimplant it here, in the tragic present, she knows she has to do it, and when she finally manages to express herself, she is neither concrete nor precise, she's incoherent, so much so that he begins to lose his calm, he too seized by terror – something has happened, something bad – and Sean starts questioning her, infuriated, is it Simon? what about Simon? what about surfing? an accident where? Within the texture of sound his face appears, precise as in the photo onscreen. She imagines he might deduce a drowning, corrects herself, the monosyllables becoming sentences that slowly organise and form meaning, and soon she drops into order everything she knows, closing her eyes and placing the phone flat against her sternum at the sound of Sean's scream. Then gathering herself again, she quickly specifies that yes, the condition is life-threatening, that he's in a coma but is still alive, and Sean, disfigured in his turn, disfigured as she is, answers I'm coming, I'll be there in two minutes, where are you? – and his voice has changed camps now, it has joined Marianne, it has pierced the fragile membrane that separates those who are happy from those who are damned: wait for me.

Marianne finds the strength to tell him the name of the café, the umpteenth Balto in the port city, she tells him where it is – it was pouring rain the first time she came here, that was in October, four months ago, she was working on an article commissioned by the heritage foundation, had wanted to see the Church of Saint Joseph again, Oscar Niemeyer's *Volcan*, the model apartment of a Perret building, all this concrete whose movement and radical form she liked, but her notebook had got drenched and once she was at the bar, streaming, she had downed a whisky, straight: Sean had started sleeping at the hangar, he had left the apartment, taking nothing with him.

She makes out her form in the mirror at the back, then her face, the one he will see after all this time, after this heaping up of silence; she has imagined this moment for a long time, promising herself that she will be so beautiful when it comes, beautiful as she still can be, and that he will be dazzled if not touched, but now dried tears have stretched her skin and it's dry as though covered with a clay mask, and her swollen lids only weakly ventilate the pale pale green he likes to plumb.

She empties the glass of gin in one gulp, and then he's there, standing before her, haggard and ravaged; bits of wood dusting his hair, sticking in the folds of his clothes and the creases of his sweater. She gets up, a sudden movement, her chair topples over – clatters to the ground – but she doesn't turn, stands facing him, one hand flat against the table to support her shaking body, the other hanging at her side – they look at each other for a fraction of a second and then with one step they're embracing, an embrace with a crazy force, as though they were crushing themselves into one another, heads pressed together hard enough to split open, shoulders compressed beneath the mass of thoraxes, arms hurting from holding on so hard they intermingle scarves, vests and coats; the kind of embrace you give in order to become a rock in the cyclone, a stone before leaping into the void, like something from the end of the world while at the same time, at the exact same time, it's also a gesture that reconnects them – their lips touch – that underlines and does away with the distance, and when they disincarcerate each other, when they finally release each other, stunned, done in, they're like sailors washed up after a shipwreck.

*

Once they're sitting down, Sean sniffs Marianne's glass. Gin? Marianne smiles – clowning – points to the menu on the wall and begins to read aloud all the things he could order for lunch this Sunday, for example a croque-monsieur, croque-madame, Perigord salad, haddock and potatoes, plain omelette, tartine provençale, fried sausages, crème caramel, crème vanilla, apple tart, and if she could she would read the whole chalkboard out to him and keep reading in a loop in order to delay the moment when she would have to put it back on, the costume of the bird of ill omen, those feathers of darkness and tears. He lets her go on, watches her without a word, and then gives in to impatience and grabs her by the wrist, his hand cuffing the slender joint and compressing the artery, please, stop. He, too, orders a gin.

Then Marianne arms herself with courage – arms herself, yes, that's exactly it, there is this naked aggression that hasn't stopped growing since their embrace and which she covers herself with now, the way we protect ourselves by brandishing the blade of the dagger – and, from the bench seat, direct, delivers the three propositions she had prepared – her eyes stare straight ahead. When he hears the last one – "irreversible" – Sean shakes his head and his face twists, convulses, no, no, no, and he gets up, heavy, bumps against the table – the gin spills over the rim of the glass – heads for the door, arms at his sides and fists tight as though he were carrying a weight, the bearing of a man who's going out to break someone's face, who's looking for him already, and when he gets to the doorstep outside he turns abruptly, comes back to the table, moving through the ray of light traced on the ground, and his backlit silhouette is haloed with a greyish powder: the sawdust that covers him lifts into space each time his foot hits the ground. His body smokes. And he's storming forward, chest inclined as though he were about to charge. Once he reaches the table he grabs the glass of gin and, like her, empties it in one gulp, then shoots at Marianne, who's already knotting her scarf, let's go.

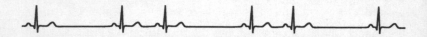

THE ROOM IS BATHED IN HALF-LIGHT, THE GROUND REFLECTS A curdled sky between the blinds, and, as a result, you have to let your eyes adjust before being able to make out the machines, the furniture, and the body that inhabits it. Simon Limbeau is there, stretched out on his back in a bed, a white sheet pulled up to his chest. He's hooked up to a respirator. The sheet rises slightly with each inhalation, a small but perceptible movement – you might say he was sleeping. The murmur of the ward is muffled, and the constant vibrations of the medical equipment only emphasise the silence as they bore into it with their *basso continuo*. This could be the room of someone who was sick, yes, you could believe this, if it weren't for the dimness, subdued, and the sense of withdrawal, as though this room were actually somewhere outside the hospital, a depressurised alveolus where nothing more takes place.

They don't say anything in the car, nothing, there is nothing to say yet. Sean had left his car parked in front of the bar – a station wagon running out of steam stuffed full of skiffs he's made, and the surfboards that Simon has collected, gathered from here and there, shortboards or fishes – and got into Marianne's car, a first, where she drove with forearms parallel and stiff as matchsticks while he kept his face turned toward the window, from time to time uttering some commentary about the traffic's smooth flow – a flow that was their ally, carrying them quickly to their son's bedside, but a flow that was also, from the first rings of the telephone, pushing them quickly toward calamity without any possibility of avoidance: nothing came to hinder or slow them on their path toward the hospital. Of course, the chance of a twist came to both their minds at the same moment – scanner results presented backwards, a mix-up in the scans, a mistake in the reading, a typing error, a computer bug, it could happen, yes, just like two babies can sometimes be switched in the maternity ward, or like times when the patient brought to the O.R. isn't the one waiting for an operation, hospitals aren't infallible – without either of them being able completely to believe it, and without them being able to say it openly to one another, and then buildings with smooth windowed facades grew under their gazes until they engulfed the windshield, and now they were groping around in this room.

Marianne goes over to Simon, as near as possible to this body that has never seemed so long before, and that she hasn't seen up this close for years – Simon's modesty, locked in the bathroom, demanding that they knock before coming into his room, or walking through the apartment draped in towels like a young *bonze*. Marianne leans over her child's mouth to feel his breath, places a cheek against his chest to hear his heart. He's breathing, she can feel it; his heart is beating, she can hear it – does she think then of the first heartbeats perceived at the ultrasound clinic at the Odeon in Paris one autumn afternoon, the first cavalcade of rapid beats when spots of light amassed on the screen? She stands up. Simon's head is encircled by a bandage, the skin is intact, yes, but is his face still there? The question assails her as she examines her child's forehead, the slope of it, the lines of his eyebrows, the shape of his eyes beneath their lids – the little hollow of skin in the inner corner of the eye, smooth and concave – as she recognises the strong nose, the finely drawn full lips, the recess of the cheeks, the chin covered in a fine beard, yes, all of this is here, but Simon's face, all that lives and thinks within him, all that animates him, will any of that come back? She sways, legs weak, clutches the edge of the wheeled bed, the drip moves, space reels around her. Sean's outline grows blurred as though behind a windowpane spattered with raindrops. He has moved to the other side of the bed, stands directly across from Marianne, and now he takes his son's hand while from the frozen deeps of his belly to the edge of his lips, just parted, his name is barely formed: Simon. We're here, we're with you, can you hear me, Simon, my boy, we're here. He places his forehead against that of the young man stretched out, his skin is still warm and there it is, his smell, smell of wool and cotton, smell of the sea, and Sean probably begins to whisper words just for the two of them, words that no one else can hear and that we will never know, archaic babble from the Polynesian isles, or *mana* words that have crossed unaltered through all the layers of language, embers that glow red with a fire intact, this dense, slow matter, inexhaustible, this wisdom; it lasts two or three minutes and then he stands again, his eyes meet Marianne's and their hands brush together above their child's chest, a movement that makes the sheet slip down, revealing the Maori tattoo they've never touched, vegetal design beginning at the shoulder and spreading over the indent of the clavicle and on to the shoulder blades – Simon had marked his skin in the summer of his fifteenth year at a surf camp in the Basque country, a way of stating my body is my own, and while Sean, calm, himself with tattoos across his back, had asked him about the meaning, the choice and the placement of such a design, trying to tease out whether he was giving a nod to the traces of Maori in his blood, Marianne, for her part, had taken it badly, Simon was so young, she had said, anxious, your tattoo, you know it's there for life, right? And the word comes back to her like a boomerang: irreversible.

Revol has just entered the room. Sean turns and says: I hear his heart beating – it seems like the hum of the machines grows amplified in that moment – and then again, insistent: his heart is beating, right? Yes, Revol asserts, his heart is beating, thanks to the machines. And after a moment, when he's getting ready to leave the room, Sean stops him again: why wasn't he operated on as soon as he arrived? The doctor detects the aggressive tension, the despair that's turning to anger and on top of it the father has been drinking, he smells alcohol on his breath, and he explains carefully: it wasn't possible to operate, sir, the haemorrhage was too severe, too advanced, the scan ordered in emergency when Simon was admitted clearly shows that it was too late. Maybe it's this certitude maintained in the cataclysm, this imperturbable calm approaching arrogance even while the tremors intensify, but Sean suddenly raises his voice, explodes: you didn't even try! Revol winces but doesn't bat an eye, would like to reply but feels that all he can do is remain silent, and anyway someone is knocking at the door now, and without waiting for a response Cordelia Owl enters the room.

The young woman has splashed a little water on her face, had a coffee, she's beautiful as some girls are after a sleepless night. She greets Marianne and Sean with a furtive smile and then, focused, approaches the bed. I'm going to take your temperature now. She's talking to Simon. Revol freezes. Marianne and Sean open their eyes wide, astonished. The young woman turns her back to them, murmurs, there, that's good, then she checks his blood pressure on the monitor and says, I'm going to check your catheter now, to see if you've gone pee – she moves with an almost excruciating gentleness. Revol catches the stunned look that passes between Marianne and Sean Limbeau, hesitates to interrupt the nurse, to give her the order to leave, and finally opts for movement: we need to speak in my office, please, come with me. Marianne starts, resists, doesn't want to leave the room, I'm staying with Simon – locks of hair hang in her face, accompanying the to and fro of her head that sways in the void – and Sean begins to pace with her while Revol insists, come with me, your son needs care, you can come back to see him right after.

Once again the labyrinth, corridors that break off into other corridors, once again forms of people at work, the echo, the wait, drips checked, treatments dispensed, blood pressures taken, care administered – sponge baths, bedsores – rooms aired out, sheets changed, floors washed, and once again Revol and his lanky stride, once again the panels of his white coat that glide out behind him, the minuscule office and the icy chairs, once again the swivelling chair and sulphide tipped out into the hollow of a palm at the very instant when Thomas Remige knocks at the door and, without waiting, strides into the room, introduces himself to Simon Limbeau's parents, states his profession – I'm a nurse, I work on the floor – then he pulls up a stool, sits at Revol's side. So now they are four, seated in this cubbyhole, and Revol feels he has to speed things up because they're suffocating in here. He takes care to look at them each in turn, this man and this woman, Simon Limbeau's parents – once again, the gaze as a commitment to speech – while he states: Simon's brain registers no further activity, the thirty-minute electroencephalogram just taken shows a flatline – Simon is now in an irreversible coma.

Pierre Revol has gathered up his body, hollowed out his back, and stretched out his neck, a contraction of muscles as though he were shifting into higher gear, as though he were urging himself on in this moment – okay, let's cut the formalities, we have to keep moving, and it is probably this muscular focus that allows him to get past Marianne's shudder and Sean's exclamation, who recognise together the word "irreversible", understanding that the conclusion is near, and the imminence of the announcement is completely unbearable. Sean closes his lids, leans his head forward, pinches the inner corner of his eyes between thumb and forefinger and murmurs I want to be sure that everything has been done, and Revol, gentle, assures him: the impact of the accident was too violent, Simon's condition was hopeless when he was admitted this morning, we transmitted the scan to expert neurosurgeons who, unfortunately, confirmed that a surgical intervention couldn't fix anything, you have my word. He says "condition was hopeless" and the parents stare at the ground. Inside them, everything cracks and caves in and suddenly, as though to delay the final word, Marianne says: yes, but people wake up from comas, it happens that they wake up, even years later, there are tons of cases like that, right? Her face is transfigured at this idea, a flash of light, and her eyes grow wide, yes, with a coma, nothing is ever sure, she knows it, stories abound of people who wake up after years, they fill up blogs, forums, these miraculous stories. Revol stops her eyes with his own, and replies, firm: no – the syllable that kills. He starts again: the functions of relational life, in other words, your son's consciousness, sensibility and mobility are non-existent, and even his vegetative functions, his breathing and blood circulation are only happening because of machines – Revol unfurls, unfurls, as though he were proceeding by accumulation of evidence, his words enumerate, pause after each piece of information, while the intonation lifts, a way of saying that bad news piles up, that it heaps up within Simon's body, until his sentence wears itself out, finally stops, suddenly indicating the emptiness stretched out before it, like a dissolution of space.

– Simon is brain-dead. Deceased. He's dead.

One needs time, of course, to catch one's breath after uttering such a thing, time to take a pause, stabilise the oscillations of the inner ear so as not to collapse in a heap on the ground. Gazes dissolve. Revol ignores the beep beep at his belt, opens his hand, studies the orangey paperweight growing warm against his palm. He's sucked dry. He just told this man and this woman that their son is dead, didn't clear his throat, didn't lower his voice, said the words, the word "deceased", and, worse still, the word "dead", these words that freeze a bodily state. But Simon Limbeau's body is not frozen, that is exactly the problem, and his aspect contravenes the usual idea of a corpse: it is, after all, warm, flushed, and it moves – rather than being cold, blue and immobile.

Slanting the angle of his eyes, Revol observes Marianne and Sean – she burns her irises on the yellow fluorescent tube attached to the ceiling, while he rests his forearms on his thighs, face tilted toward the ground, head sunk between his shoulders – what might they have seen in their son's room? what might they have understood, with their untrained eyes, when they couldn't make the link between Simon's destroyed interior and his peaceful exterior, between the inside and the outside? Their child's body offered no evidence, manifested no physical sign that would allow the diagnosis to be made from a reading of the body – you might think of the fantastic "Babinski reflex", capable of detecting diseases of the brain simply via stimulation of the sole of the foot – for them it lay undecipherable, mute, closed as a chest. Remige's phone rings, sorry, he leaps to his feet and shuts it off, sits down again, Marianne sits shaking beside Sean who doesn't lift his head, unmoving, his back wide, rounded, black.

Revol keeps them in his field of vision, he surrounds them, his gaze like a lens scanning over their movements, these two are a little younger than him, children from the late 1960s, they live in a part of the world where life expectancy just keeps getting higher, where we're shielded from a view of death, where it's erased from the day-to-day, carried off to the hospital where it's handled by professionals. Have they even seen a corpse before? Watched over a grandmother, found a drowned person, sat with a friend as she neared the end of life? Have they seen a dead person other than on an American T.V. series, *Body of Proof, CSI, Six Feet Under*? Revol likes to stroll from time to time through these televisual morgues, where emergency doctors, medical examiners, undertakers, embalmers, and hotshot forensic teams meander amid a good number of sexy, frenzied girls – usually some gothic creature flaunting a tongue piercing left and right or a girlfriend who's classy but bipolar, always thirsty for love – he likes listening to this little world chattering away around a stiff stretched out across the bluish screen, confiding in each other, flirting shamelessly – even working, formulating hypotheses from a single hair brandished at the end of a pair of tweezers, a button under the micro-scope, a swab of oral mucus analysed up close, because the clock is always ticking, the night always has to come to an end, because it's always urgent that they elucidate the traces recorded in the epider-mis, try their hand at deciphering flesh that can tell us whether the victim went to nightclubs, sucked lozenges, ate too much red meat, drank whisky, was afraid of the dark, dyed his hair, worked with chemicals, had sex with multiple partners; yes, Revol sometimes likes to watch these episodes, even though, in his opinion, the series don't say anything about death, the corpse may well fill the focal range, asphyxiate the screen, be scrutinised, fractioned, turned over, but it's only a simulacra, and everything unfolds as though, as long as it hasn't revealed all its secrets, as long as it remains a potentiality – nar-rative, dramaturgical – this corpse could keep death at a distance.

Sean and Marianne still haven't made a single movement. Despair, bravery, dignity, Revol doesn't know, was just as ready to see them explode, come hurtling over his desk, send his papers flying, knock over his stupid ornaments, even hit and yell at him – bastard, shithead – there is enough reason to come unhinged, to bash their heads against the wall, scream their rage, instead of which, everything was happening as though these two were slowly dissociating them-selves from the rest of humanity, migrating toward the edges of the earth's crust, leaving a time and a territory behind to begin a sidereal drift.

How could they even conceive of the death of their child, when this absolute – death, the most pure of all absolutes – had been reshaped, rewritten, into different bodily states? Because it was no longer this rhythm beating in the hollow of the chest that confirmed life – a soldier removes his helmet and leans down to place an ear on the chest of his comrade lying in the mud at the bottom of the trench – it is no longer the breath exhaled through the mouth that indicates life – water streams off an expert swimmer as she performs mouth-to-mouth on a young girl with a greenish complexion – but rather the brain electrified, activated by cerebral waves, beta waves preferably. How could they even envision it, Simon's death, when his complexion still flushes pink, and supple, when his nape still bathes in cool blue watercress and he's stretched out with his feet in the gladiolus. Revol rounds up the paintings of corpses that he knows, and they're always images of Christ, Christs on the cross with pallid bodies, foreheads scratched by the crown of thorns, feet and hands nailed to shining black wood, or Christs deposed, heads back and eyelids half-closed, deathly pale, scrawny, hips girdled with a thin swaddling like in a Mantegna, or Holbein the Younger's *Body of the Dead Christ in the Tomb* – a painting of such incredible realism that Dostoyevsky warned believers against it: looking at it, they risked losing their faith – or the dead are kings, prelates, embalmed dictators, those movie cowboys collapsed on the sand and filmed close up, and he remembers then that photo of Che, Christlike, indeed, he too with eyes open, laid out in a morbid staging by the Bolivian junta, but he can't think of anything that would be analogous to Simon, to this intact body, to this unbleeding body, calmly athletic, like a young god at rest, that seems to be sleeping, that seems to be alive.

How long did they stay sitting like that after the words were pronounced, slumped at the edge of their chairs, gripped by a mental experience their bodies couldn't even have imagined before? How long would it take them to accept their place under death's regime? For the moment, there is no possible translation for what they feel – it strikes them down into a language that precedes language, an unshareable language, before words and before grammar, which may be the other name for pain, they can't escape it, they can't describe nor form any image of it, they are at once cut off from themselves and cut off from the world.

Thomas Remige has remained silent on the metal stool beside Revol, legs crossed, and maybe he's been thinking of the same things, maybe he's been forming the same scenes. He's put away his box of matches, and waits with them, time ticks on, brains to pulp and mute screams, and then Revol stands, towering and pallid, his long face full of desolation indicating that he has to leave the room, I have to go, and Thomas Remige stays alone with the Limbeaus who don't get up but lean in close to each other, shoulder to shoulder, and cry silently. He waits a moment and then asks them in a voice full of care if they want to go back to Simon's room. They stand up without answering, the nurse falling into step behind them, but once they are in the corridor Sean shakes his head, no, I don't want to go back, I can't, not right away, he's breathing hard, lungs inflating and chest lifting, hand to his mouth, Marianne slips under his shoulder – to support him, to protect herself – and the trio stops moving forward. Thomas comes nearer and says: I'm here for you, here to assist you; if you have any questions, please ask. Sean staggers, and then – how does he find the strength to articulate it? – says all at once: what's going to happen now? The nurse swallows while Sean goes on, voice ravaged by grief and revolt: why is he being kept in intensive care if there's no hope? What are they waiting for? I don't understand. Marianne, her hair in her face, her eyes staring, stricken, seems not to hear anything, while Thomas searches for a way out, an answer he can formulate: Sean's question interrupts the protocol's timeline, which had been formulated to counter the speed of the tragedy and the violence of the news, to stretch out time, if we could just have some time. It's a cry that he must answer. He decides to speak to them now.

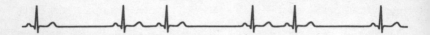

CORDELIA OWL PLUMPS UP THE PILLOW AROUND SIMON'S HEAD, smooths the sheet over his chest, draws the curtains, pulls the door of the room closed behind her, and walks to the department front desk, tracing arabesques in the hallway – damn these stiff, tight-fitting scrubs, she would have liked something roomier in this moment, to hear the rasping of pleats, to feel them brush against her bumpy knees that she knows are supple and clever. On the way, she plunges her hand into her pocket, pulls out her mobile: no message. Nothing. *Nada de nada.* 2.40 p.m. He must be sleeping, he's sleeping. He's stretched out somewhere on his back, chest bare, abandoned. She smiles. Don't call.

Reknickered, rebuttoned, belt buckles readjusted, they had faced each other on the pavement, well, well, I'm gonna go, yeah it's late, um, you mean early, yeah, okay bye, bye, a kiss on the cheek, a kind smile, then, following the appropriate adage, they separated – smooth balancé, dégagé to the back, piqué turn – moving away along the same line before each melted into the darkness. Cordelia had walked slowly at first, letting her heels resonate like a starlet from the 1950s in a tight pencil skirt, the collar of her coat held tight by a hand pressed to her throat, she hadn't turned around, she wouldn't, but once she'd rounded the corner she tipped her head up to the sky and spun around wind in her mouth, arms out horizontal like a whirling dervish, then falling into line again had continued on her course, rushing quickly along city blocks, from time to time daring a large jeté over a gutter as though it were a river she had to ford, and her arms undulated like ribbons, the cold of the night whipped at her face, the icy air dove in between the front flaps of her coat, open wide at that moment, and it was good, she felt beautiful, supple, taller by at least twenty centimetres since they had clattered against garbage cans, since her underwear had fallen to the ground and he had placed a perfectly hollowed palm between her legs to lift her up against the wall, since she had stood up on one tiptoe, had bent the knee of her other leg to her chest, pulling him toward her now, inside her, tongues monopolising mouths like the fire the oven, teeth eventually biting, she laughed her way home, hot—cold girl who's been around the block, overplaying the solitary heroine to the eyes of the world, Amazon of the city taking her desire in hand, master of her actions, she walked along the windy boulevards, the frozen streets of five in the morning, raced along, indifferent to the car that slowed beside her, to the windows that lowered to let a sexual insult spurt out, want a ride, bitch? she devoured space, a combustion, and so she was almost crossing rue Étretat when Chris's van changed lanes on her left at the Quatre-Chemins intersection, slammed on the brakes at the edge of the pavement, the fresco of the body of the van displayed before her – it seemed to her that the Californian surfers in triangle bikinis were giving her the eye and smiling, as at a potential sister – and a few strides later she was at her place, buried under the feather duvet, eyes closed but she couldn't fall asleep, she hadn't asked anything of this guy who'd tormented her for aeons, hadn't asked a single question – brave girl.

She goes into the office, windowed like an aquarium, a chair, she collapses into it. Totally drained. Clownfish criss-cross the computer screen. She probes her phone again. Zilch. *Nada*, of course. A tacit sign she won't transgress. Not for all the gold in the world. The idea that, even if it were said in a fast voice and a cool tone, the smallest word couldn't be anything but false, heavy, viscous, and the least sentence would reveal her anxiety under the false bottom, sentimental twit. Don't move a finger, toss back a coffee, dried fruits, a vial of royal jelly, don't do anything stupid, turn off the phone. God I'm exhausted.

Pierre Revol comes in while she's examining the purple traces on her neck, contorting herself before the Photo Booth app, and seeing his face appear in the picture, leaning over her shoulder like a nosy reader taking advantage of his neighbour's newspaper in the Metro, she lets out a yelp. You're new in the department, you said? Revol stands still behind her as she leaps up, spins around, dizzy, black veil before her eyes, I should eat something, she tucks her hair behind her ears again, a way of clearing a space on her unstable face, yes, I started two days ago, and with a firm hand she readjusts the collar of her uniform. There's something important I need to talk to you about, something you'll be confronted with here. Cordelia nods her head, okay, now? It won't take long, it's about what just happened in the room, but right at that moment, bzzz, bzzz, Cordelia's phone vibrates at the bottom of her pocket and here she is holding herself as though she's getting an electric shock, oh no, no, unbelievable, shit! Revol has leaned against the back of a chair and he starts talking, head tilted toward the ground, arms crossed over his chest, and legs crossed too at the ankle, the boy you saw is brain-dead, bzzz, bzzz, Revol expresses himself distinctly, but to Cordelia his words sound like a phonetics exercise in a foreign language – even if she channelled all the attention she's capable of toward this face and kept her brain focused on this voice talking, still everything is happening as though she were swimming against the current, against this hot wave that seeps along the length of her hip at regular intervals, bzzz, bzzz, drips into the fold of her thigh, into the hollow of her groin, she fights against it, tries to come back, but Revol gets further and further away, as though he'd tumbled into the rapids, and becomes less and less audible as he explains: so you see, this young man is dead; comprehending the reality of his death is difficult for those close to him, and the way his body looks confuses this fact, do you understand? Cordelia tries hard to listen, articulates a yes like you might pop a bubble, I see, but she doesn't see anything, the birdbrain, in fact it's a stampede in her brain, bzzz, bzzz, the infinitesimal tremors of the telephone now carrying their lot of sexual images, photograms lifted from the film of the night before – there's that incredibly soft mouth open on her neck and that hot breath as her forehead, her cheek, her belly, now her breasts graze the wall, red from scraping the grainy mortar and the jutting stones with him behind her, and her hands grabbed his buttocks to bring him closer still, deeper and harder – bzzz, last flutter, it's over, she doesn't blink, swallows before answering in a stiff voice yes, I understand completely, so that Revol tosses her a kindly look before concluding, okay: so when you're doing the rounds, you can't speak to a patient who's brain-dead the way you did, his parents were in the room and for them that was a contradictory sign in an extreme situation, talking like that during a check-up muddles the message we're trying to give them, the situation is already so difficult, are we on the same page? Yes – Cordelia's voice, tortured, waiting for one thing and one thing only – for Revol to take off, go on get out, get out now, I get it, and suddenly, though there was no warning, she digs her heels in, lifts her head: you didn't involve me in the patient's intake, you saw his parents alone, we don't work like that anymore. Revol looks at her, surprised: oh? And how do we work then? Cordelia takes a step forward and slaps down her reply: we work as a team. Silence stretches out, they look at each other, then the doctor stands up straight: you're looking quite pale, have you been shown the kitchen? There are cookies in there, watch yourself, twelve hours in the I.C.U. is a marathon, young lady, you have to be able to go the distance. Yes, okay, okay. Revol finally agrees to leave the room, and Cordelia plunges her hand into her pocket. She closes her eyes, thinks of her grandmother in Bristol whom she speaks to every Sunday evening, it's not her, it's not the right time for her she says to convince herself, would have gladly hazarded a guess before lifting her lids and reading the numbers inscribed on the little touch screen, would gladly bet, as in a roulette game, on a room number that lights up on the board, would try to throw a paper ball in a bin or simply play heads or tails with a coin – don't be such a silly goose, what's your problem?

Cordelia Owl goes to stand in the middle of the room, lifts her head, and throws shoulders back, slowly opens her fingers, revealing phalanx after phalanx the number that called her. Unknown. She smiles, relieved. In the end, not so entirely certain that she wants it to happen, not in such a hurry to hear from him. She's suddenly cruel, when she thinks of him, she's lucid and laughing. She's twenty-eight years old. Anticipates with disgust the exhaustion of romantic tension, that mountain of exhaustion – exaltation, anxiety, craziness, crass impulsiveness – asks herself again why this intensity continues to be the most desirable part of her life, but then whirls around, turns away from this question the way you pull the tip of your toe back at the very last moment from the sludgy pond where it was about to land, to sink, she never gets any peace, what she needs is to prolong last night, let it steep like the afterglow of a party. Conserve the grace and the irony of girls. Once she reaches the small kitchen, she takes a pack of raspberry cookies from the cupboard, pulls open the paper that squeaks like silk under her little fingers, slowly and completely devours the pack.

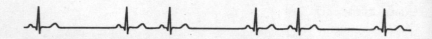

REVOL WALKS BACK DOWN THE HALL, IGNORING THOSE WHO call out and scamper along beside him, holding out forms, three minutes, dammit, he mutters between his teeth, I just want three minutes, thumb, index, and middle finger held up in the air while his voice stresses "three", and the department staff know this gesture well, know that once he's alone in his office the anaesthetist will gravitate toward the chair that sways and rolls, look at his watch, and start a countdown – three minutes, a soft-boiled egg, the ideal measure – and using this lapse of solitude as a kind of decompression chamber, will place his cheek on his forearm folded flat against the desk, exactly the way children in kindergarten nap in the classroom after snack time – and will dive into this crevice of rest to stem the tide of what's just happened, might even fall asleep. Wiped out, he rests his head on his folded arms and dozes off. Everyone understands that he makes the most of these three minutes: after so many years of putting others to sleep (twenty-seven), you'd have to have refined a technique of high-efficiency micro-napping, even if the duration were slightly inferior to what was generally advised for recharging a human body. Everyone knows that Revol lost that other sleep long ago, the nocturnal, the horizontal, the deep sleep. In the apartment he occupies on rue de Paris there isn't even really a bedroom anymore, just a large room with a double bed that serves as a coffee table, that's where he keeps his record collection – all of Bob Dylan and Neil Young – piles of paper, and long trays where psychotropic plants grow, his botanical experiments – it's professional, he says to the few who drop by, surprised to see cannabis plants growing right out in the open, as well as opium and common poppies, lavender and *Salvia divinorum*, the "sage of the seers", a hallucinogenic herb whose curative virtues he has described in articles published in pharmacology journals.

The night before, alone in his apartment, he watched Paul Newman's film *The Effect of Gamma Rays on Man-in-the-Moon Marigolds* for the first time – the title indeed suggested a botanical fantasy, but it was powerful in a totally different way, a film that traced a path between hallucination and science, and it had captivated Revol right from the start. Stirred, taken in, he had the bud of an idea – why not – to reproduce the young heroine's experiment in his own living room. Matilda had subjected marigolds to different doses of radium in order to observe their growth, their shapes that became differentiated after several days under the influence of the rays, some of them becoming enormous, others scrawny and wrinkled, still others simply beautiful, and bit by bit this solitary girl began to understand something of the infinite variety of the living, at the same time that she was coming to take her place in the world, proclaiming aloud, on the theatre stage after the school festival, the possibility that a marvellous mutation could one day transform and improve the whole human race. After which, deep in thought, he fried some eggs sunny side up, their yellows as brilliant as the marigolds' hearts, uncapped a light beer pulled from the door of the fridge, slowly swallowed all of it, then rolled himself in a goose-down duvet, eyes wide open.

Revol sleeps. A notebook lies within arm's reach so that he can jot things down when he wakes, describe the images glimpsed, the actions, sequences, and faces, and maybe Simon's face will be among them – the black locks stiff with coagulated blood, the olive, tumid skin, the white domes of the eyelids, the forehead and right temple swallowed up by a beet-red ring, the mortal macula – or maybe it will be Joanne Woodward's, alias Beatrice Hunsdorfer, Matilda's borderline mother, who suddenly surfaces in the theatre once the festival is over, emerges from the shadow in fine evening dress, sequins and black feathers, staggering, drunk, eyes glassy, and declares in a slurred voice, hand on her sternum: my heart is full, my heart is full.

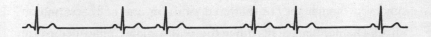

THEY HOLD HANDS AS THEY FOLLOW THOMAS REMIGE AND, IN the end, if they go with him, if they comply with this other perambulation in the latticework of corridors and airlocks, if they agree to pass through all those tide gates, to open all those doors and hold them with their shoulders, despite the black meteor that had just hit them full force, and despite their obvious exhaustion, it's probably because Thomas Remige looks upon them justly – holds them in a gaze that keeps them on the side of the living, a gaze that is already infinitely precious. And so, along the way, these two interlace fingers, touch chewed finger pads, bitten nails edged with dead skin, brush dry palms together, rings and stones, and they do it without even thinking.

This is yet another area of the hospital, a hideout decorated like the living room of a model apartment: the room is bright, the furniture smart but ordinary – an apple-green couch in synthetic fabric that feels like velvet and two vermilion chairs with puffy cushions – the walls bare except for a colour poster from a Kandinsky exhibit – Beaubourg, 1985 – and, placed on the surface of the low table, a green plant with long thin leaves, four clean glasses, a bottle of mineral water, and a small dish of potpourri scented with orange and cinnamon. The window is half-open, the curtains sway lightly, you can hear the sound of the occasional car come and go in the hospital parking lot and, like sonorous scratches over everything, the stridence of gulls. It's cold.

Sean and Marianne sit side by side on the couch, awkward, curious even though they're shattered, and, on one of the vermilion chairs Thomas Remige sits down too, with Simon Limbeau's medical folder in his hands. But even though these three share the same space, participate in the same time period, nothing on this planet could be further apart than these two beings in pain and this young man who sits before them with the goal – yes, the goal – of obtaining their consent to recover their child's organs. On one side: a man and a woman caught in a wave of shock, at once swept off the ground and crashed down into a dislocated timeline – a continuity that Simon's death had ruptured, but a continuity that, like a headless duck running in a farmyard, continued on – total madness – a timeline woven of pain, a man and a woman gathering all the sorrow of the world upon their two heads, and on the other side: this young man in a white lab coat – committed and cautious, prepared to conduct the meeting without skipping any steps, but who has set a timer in a corner of his brain, conscious that once brain death occurs, the body deteriorates rapidly, and that this has to be done quickly – caught in the same torsion.

Thomas pours water into the glasses, gets up to close the window, crosses the room, and as he does so watches this couple, doesn't let his eyes leave them for a second, this man and this woman, Simon Limbeau's parents, and at this moment he's probably warming up mentally, aware that he's gearing up for some rough treatment, to make an incision in their grief and insert a question of which they are as yet unaware, to ask them to reflect and to form answers, when they are zombies hard-hit by pain, satellited; and he's probably preparing to talk to them the way he prepares himself to sing, relaxing his muscles, regulating his breathing, conscious that punctuation is the anatomy of language, the structure of meaning, and he visualises the opening sentence, its musical line, and gauges the first syllable he will utter, the one that will cleave the silence, precise, rapid as a cut – more like a gash than the crack in the eggshell or the lizard that climbs the wall when the earth quakes. He begins slowly, methodically restating the context of the situation: I think you understand that Simon's brain damage is irreversible, and yet his organs continue to function; it's an exceptional situation. Sean and Marianne blink their eyes, a kind of agreement. Thomas, encouraged, continues: I'm conscious of the pain you must be in, but I have to broach a sensitive subject with you – his face is enshrouded in a transparent light and his voice rises a notch imperceptibly, absolutely clear when he says:

– This is a situation where it would be possible to imagine Simon as an organ donor.

Bam. From the beginning, Thomas had tuned his voice to the right frequency and the room seems to vibrate like a giant microphone, a high-precision strike – wheels of the Rafale jet on the flight deck of the aircraft carrier, Japanese calligrapher's brush, tennis player's drop shot. Sean lifts his head, Marianne starts, both their gazes spill into Thomas's own – they begin to glimpse with terror what's happening here, sitting before this handsome young man with the medallion profile, this handsome young man who continues calmly. I wanted to ask if your son had had the chance to express his views on the subject, if he had ever spoken to you about it.

The walls waltz, the ground rolls, Marianne and Sean are bowled over. Speechless, gazes floating level with the low table, hands twisting, and this silence that spills, thick, dark, vertiginous, panic mixed with confusion. A void has opened up before them, a void that they can't imagine other than as "something" because "nothing" is simply unthinkable. They struggle against this gaping hole in the air, together, even though the questions and emotions that shake them are not the same – Sean has become, over the years, solitary and of few words, combining the most clear non-belief with a lyrical spirituality, drawn from Oceanian myths, whereas Marianne was a first communicant in a flowered dress and tennis socks, forehead banded with a crown of fresh flowers and the host stuck to the roof of her mouth, who prayed for a long time in the evenings in the bunk bed she shared with her sister, kneeling in the top bunk, speaking her praise aloud in her scratchy pyjamas, and still today she enters churches, explores the silence there like the texture of a mystery, looks for the little red light behind the altar, inhales the heavy scent of wax and incense, observes the light of day filtered by the rosette in coloured rays, the wooden statues with their painted eyes, but remembers the intense sensation that rushed through her in the moment when she removed the yoke of faith; both of them see visions of death in the air, images of the beyond, post-mortem spaces plunged into eternity: it's a chasm tucked inside a fold of the cosmos, it's a black and wrinkled lake, it's the realm of the believers, a garden where, beneath the hand of God, beings with resuscitated flesh come back to life, it's a lost valley in the jungle where forsaken souls flutter about, it's a desert of ash, a sleep, a detour, a Dantesque hole at the bottom of the sea, and it's also an unreproducible coast that you reach in a delicately crafted wooden dugout. They're leaning forward, arms crossed over abdomens to absorb the shock, and their thoughts converge into a funnel of questions they can't formulate.

Thomas starts again – takes another tack – did your son register his refusal to become a donor with the national database? Or do you know if he expressed any opposition to the idea, if he was against it? Complicated sentence, their faces distort. Marianne shakes her head, I don't know, I don't think so, she stammers, and Sean suddenly becomes animated, his face weathered and square, turns slowly toward Thomas and says, carving through space with a hollow voice: nineteen years old – with these poorly articulated words, emitted through tight lips, his chest sways forward, imposing – are there any nineteen-year-old boys who make arrangements about this, for . . . do they exist? – "make arrangements": he raises his voice, submachine guns the velar consonants, an icy fire. It can happen, Thomas replies gently, it's sometimes the case. Sean takes a gulp of water, puts the glass down heavily: maybe, but not Simon. Then, sidling into what he identifies as a gap in the dialogue, Thomas asks, raising his voice a notch, why "not Simon"? Sean looks at him hard, spits out: because he loves life so much. Thomas nods, I understand, but keeps on: loving live doesn't mean he wouldn't have imagined death, he might have spoken about it to some of the people close to him. Filaments of silence that converge, splice together, and then Marianne reacts, misty and quick: people close to him, yes, I don't know, if, his sister, yes, he loves his little sister a lot, Lou, she's seven, they're like cat and dog but they're lost without each other, and his friends, yes, for sure, his surfing friends, Johan, Christophe, his friends from school, yes, I don't

97

know, I think so, we don't see them that often, but the people close to him, I don't know exactly who they are, well yes his grandmother, his cousin who lives in the States, and there's Juliette too, Juliette, his first love, yes, the people close to him, that's us.

They're speaking of their son in the present, this is not a good sign. Thomas goes on: I'm asking you these questions because if the deceased person, in this case your son Simon, didn't make his refusal known when he was living, if he didn't express consent, we have to decide together what he would have wanted – "the deceased person, in this case your son Simon," Thomas raises his voice and pronounces each word distinctly, he drives the nail in. Consent to what? It's Marianne who speaks, lifting her head – but she knows already, she wants to have the nail driven in. Thomas says: consent to organ recovery for transplants – it's necessary to get through the brutality of these sentences unfolded like slogans on banners, necessary to get through their enormous weight, their bluntness – meetings where ambiguity lingers are creels of suffering, Thomas knows.

The tension mounts all at once at this point on the earth's crust – it seems that the plant's leaves tremble and the surface of the water shivers in the glasses, and it also seems as though the light intensifies, causing them to blink, and that the air begins to vibrate as though the motor of a centrifuge were slowly starting up above their heads. Thomas is the only one to remain absolutely still, doesn't betray a single emotion, looks levelly at their faces wrung out by suffering, takes in the seismic quaking of jaws and the trembling of shoulders, dodges nothing – he continues: the aim of this meeting is to seek out and formulate what Simon would have wanted; it is not about asking yourselves what you would do, rather for us to ask what your son would have decided – Thomas holds his breath, he measures the contained violence of these last words, words that radically distinguish their bodies from that of their child, inscribe a distance, but words that simultaneously allow them to think. And Marianne asks in a weak voice, trailing: how can we know?

She's asking for a method, Sean looks at her, and Thomas answers swiftly – in that moment he tells himself that maybe Marianne is, according to the expression he acquired during a training seminar, "the resource person"; in other words, the one who could create a wake effect – we are here to think about Simon, about the person he was; the process for organ donation always refers to a single individual, to our reading of his existence; we have to reflect together; for example, we might ask whether Simon was a believer, or whether he was generous. Generous? Marianne repeats, dumbfounded. Yes, generous, Thomas confirms, how he was in his relationships with others, if he was curious, if he went travelling, these are the kinds of questions we need to ask.

Marianne casts a glance at Sean, his face is undone, earthy skin and dark lips, then her eyes veer toward the green plant. She doesn't make the link between the coordinator's questions and organ donation, and finally murmurs: Sean, was Simon generous? Eyes scurry off into their corners, they don't know what to say, breathe deeply, she puts an arm around the neck of this man with hair thick and dark like his son, pulls him toward her, their foreheads touch, and he lowers his head while a "yes" slips out of his tight throat – a "yes" that doesn't really have much to do with their son's generosity, because, truth be told, Simon wasn't all that generous, he was more of a cat, egotistical and light on his feet, grumbling with his head in the fridge shit is all the Coke gone? More like that than a young man inclined to prodigious gestures, to thoughtfulness; but a *yes* that grasps the whole of Simon, raises him up to make him shine, this reserved and direct boy who devoured the intensity of youth.

Suddenly Marianne's voice breaks through a breath and her phrasing, although halted, lights up: there is one thing, we're Catholic, Simon's been baptised. She stops short. Thomas waits for her to go on but the pause stretches out, and so he asks – a supporting wall – was he a believer? Did he believe in the resurrection of the body? Marianne looks at Sean, still sees only his inclined profile, and bites her lips, I don't know, we don't often practise. Thomas stiffens – last year, parents had refused to have any organs retrieved from their daughter's body – they believed in the resurrection of the flesh, and this mutilation would make any other form of existence impossible – and when Thomas had cited the Church's official position, favourable toward organ donation, they had remained firm: we don't want to make her die a second time. Marianne rests her head on Sean's shoulder and then starts to speak again, last summer he read that book about a Polynesian shaman, the coral man, I don't know, he planned to go and meet him there, do you remember? It was a book about reincarnation, Sean agrees with eyes closed, and adds, barely audible: to exert himself, that was something that counted for Simon, he was physical, that's it, that's how he was, alive in his body, that's how I see him, nature, in nature, he wasn't scared. Marianne takes a moment and then asks, uncertain: is that what it means to be generous? I don't know, maybe – and now she's crying.

*

They're speaking in the past, the father and the mother; they've begun the telling of it. For Thomas this is a tangible step forward, the sign that the idea of their child's death is slowly crystallising. He puts the file down on the table, places his hands flat on his thighs, opens his mouth to continue, but suddenly, though there was no way to see it coming, everything topples again, a rogue wave – Sean has stood up abruptly and is pacing back and forth across the room, agitated, saying sharply, all this talk about generosity is bullshit, I don't see how the fact of being generous or travelling gives you the right to think that he would have wanted to donate his organs, that's too easy, and if I tell you that Simon was selfish does this meeting end here? Suddenly he steps close to Thomas, murmurs in his ear: just tell us, buddy, if we're allowed to say no, that's all I want to know. Marianne, shocked, turns to him, Sean! But he doesn't hear her, has straightened up again, strides back and forth in the room, faster and faster, and finally presses his back to the window, dark and massive against the light: go ahead, tell us the truth, can we refuse or not? He breathes hard, like a bull. Thomas doesn't blink, spine straight and hands moist against the fabric of his jeans. Marianne gets up and goes to Sean, she reaches out her arms but he turns away, three steps along the wall, quick spin and he punches the plaster with all his might, the glass trembles over the Kandinsky poster; he moans, fuck, this is not happening, and turns in devastation back to Thomas, who is standing now, white as a sheet, stock-still, and says firmly: Simon's body is not a warehouse of organs you can just lay your hands on, the process stops if the interview with the family to determine the deceased's intention leads to a refusal.

*

Marianne finally takes hold of Sean's hand, that wasn't very smart she murmurs as she caresses it, as if we needed this too, she pulls him toward the couch, the couple sits down again, forms again, it's a lull, each of them swallows a glass of water, even though they're not really thirsty, but it's important to temporise, to keep moving, to come back to the frequency of a few words that are possible.

At that moment, Thomas thinks it's over. Too hard. Too complex, too violent. The mother maybe, but the father . . . No distance, everything's going too fast. Barely grasped their tragedy and already they have to conceive of organ donation. He sits down again in turn. Picks up the file from the table. Wouldn't dare insist, influence, manipulate, play the authority, wouldn't dare become the agent of some silent blackmail that is all the more weighty, all the more pressing because young, healthy donors are so rare. Will spare them, for example, from hearing that, in cases where someone is not registered with the national registry of refusals, French law holds the principle of presumed consent – will spare them from having to ask how presumed consent can be the rule when the donor is dead and cannot speak anymore, can't consent, will spare them from hearing that having said nothing while he was alive was the equivalent of saying yes, or some other version of the dubious proverb "silence signifies consent", yes, he won't mention the texts that would have so easily pulverised the meaning of this dialogue, made it a simple formality, hypocritical convention, while the law concludes this other, more complex notion that has to do with reciprocity, exchange: if each individual were a presumed potential receiver, after all, was it so illogical, so unfounded, that each person should be seen as a presumed donor after their death? From now on, he won't bring up the legal aspect unless it's to open a possible way for those who have no particular connection to the concept of organ donation, or to comfort families in their decision – the law ultimately supports them like the handrail supports the hand.

He closes Simon's file and places it flat on his knees, signalling to Sean and Marianne Limbeau that they can adjourn if they wish, leave the room. It's a refusal, it happens. You have to know how to accept it – the possibility of refusal is also the condition of donation. They must say goodbye now, shake hands. The meeting was a failure, okay, he has to accept it, Thomas has adopted the principle of absolute respect of the family's decision, and also understands this indisputable aspect – the body of the deceased is sacred for his loved ones – a way of inscribing abutments in a process that runs the risk, bolstered by the law and the shortage of organs, a way of ploughing through. His eyes sweep the walls of the room; outside the window, a bird watches. A passerine bird. Thomas is surprised to see it, wonders if Ousmane will stop by his house to feed Mazhar, the goldfinch, refuel it with clean water and organic seed, those multicoloured seeds cultivated on a balcony in Bab El Oued. He closes his eyes.

Okay, what are they going to take? Sean starts up again, head down gaze low and Thomas, surprised by the change of tack, frowns and immediately adjusts to this new tempo: they would be recovering the heart, the kidneys, the lungs, and the liver; you'll be informed of everything if you consent to the process, and your child's body will be restored – he listed the organs without wavering, with this same momentum wherein he always prefers sharp precision over the vagueness of evasion.

The heart? asks Marianne. Yes, the heart Thomas repeats. Simon's heart. Marianne's head spins. Simon's heart – little islets of blood cells meet in a tiny sac to form the initial vascular network on the seventeenth day, the pump begins on the twenty-first day (minute contractile movements that are nevertheless audible with extremely sensitive equipment, designed for cardiac embryology), blood flows into conduits as they are formed, innervating tissues, veins, tubes, and arteries, the four chambers develop, everything in place on the fiftieth day even if it's not complete yet. Simon's heart – little round abdomen that rises slightly at the bottom of a playpen; the bird of night terrors panicking inside a child's chest; the staccato drum accompanying Anakin Skywalker's destiny; the shot beneath the skin when the first wave rises up – touch my pecs he'd said to her one night, muscles tensed, monkey grimace, he was fourteen and had the new shine in his eye of the boy finding himself in his body, touch my pecs, Mum; the diastolic melting when his eyes catch Juliette at the bus stop on the maritime boulevard, striped T-shirt dress, Doc Martens and red raincoat, sketchbook tucked under her arm; holding his breath among the bubble wrap on Christmas Eve, the surfboard unwrapped in the middle of the icy workshop, opened with this mix of meticulousness and ardour, the way you open the envelope containing a love letter. The heart.

But not his eyes, they won't take his eyes, right? She stifles her cry with a palm pressed against her open mouth. Sean shudders, gasps, what? His eyes? No, never, not his eyes. His moan slowly dies in the room where Thomas has lowered his own eyes, I understand.

It's another zone of turbulence, and he shivers, swimming, he knows that the symbolic charge differs from one organ to the next – Marianne, after all, only reacted to the idea of retrieving the heart, as though removing the kidneys, the liver, or the lungs were easier to imagine, and in the same way she had refused the removal of the cornea which, like the tissues and skin, the family rarely agrees to – and understands that he must compromise, let go the rule, accept the restrictions, respect this family. This is empathy. Because Simon's eyes are not just his nervous retina, his taffeta iris, his pupil of pure black in front of the crystalline – they are also his gaze; his skin isn't just the threaded mesh of his epidermis, his porous cavities – it's his light and his touch, the living sensors of his body.

– Your child's body will be restored.

It's a promise and perhaps it's also the kibosh on this dialogue, hard to say. Restored. Thomas looks at his watch, calculates – the second thirty-minute electroencephalogram will happen in two hours – would you like to take some time alone? Marianne and Sean look at each other, nod their heads. Thomas gets up and adds, if your child is a donor, that will allow others to live, other people who are waiting for an organ. The parents pick up their coats, their bags, their gestures are slow even though they're in a hurry to get out of here now. So he won't have died for nothing then, is that it? Sean turns up the collar of his parka and looks him straight in the eye, we know, we know all that already, transplants save people, the death of one person can give life to another, but – this is Simon, this is our son, do you understand that? I do. As they pass through the door, Marianne turns, looks Thomas in the eye: we're going to get some air, we'll be back.

Alone in the room, Thomas collapses into his chair, his head topples into his hands, his fingers plunge beneath his hair, into his head, and he breathes for a long moment. He must be telling himself that it's hard, and maybe he, too, would have liked to talk, punch the walls, kick the garbage bins, break some glasses. It might be a yes, more likely a no, and, it happens – one-third of meetings end in refusal –

but for Thomas Remige, a clear refusal was worth more than a consent torn from someone in confusion, delivered with forceps, and regretted fifteen days later when people are ravaged by remorse, losing sleep and sinking in sorrow, we have to think of the living, he often says, chewing the end of a little match, we have to think of the ones left behind – on the back of his office door, he had taped a photocopied page from *Platonov*, a play he's never seen, never read, but this fragment of dialogue between Voinitzev and Triletzki, found in a newspaper left lying around at the laundromat, had made him quiver the way the child discovering his fortune quivers, a Charizard in the pack of Pokémon cards, a golden ticket in the chocolate bar. What shall we do, Nicolas? Bury the dead and mend the living.

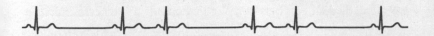

JULIETTE IS IN HER ROOM. FROM HER WINDOW, IF SHE TURNS slightly to the side and stands on tiptoe, she can see the roof of the Limbeau's building – the first time Simon came over, into her girl den, he pressed himself against the pane and then suddenly turned toward her, we can see each other, you know, and he carefully directed her gaze until she could make it out, among the marquetry of grey surfaces that stretched out below, a zinc-coloured roof strewn with chimneys where gulls were gathered: look, right there – she casts a soft eye toward it now.

They'd had a fight that night. Still, there they were, naked, lying face-to-face, squeezed together beneath warm covers, so tender that they continued to caress each other after making love, and talked to each other in the darkness, oddly voluble, their words always clearest in these moments, then the swoosh of a text had pierced the calm, and the sonar echo didn't make her laugh this time, she took it as a hostile intrusion, the surf session was on – 6.00 a.m. downstairs at your place. She didn't have to wait for him to read the message to know what it was about and to realise that he'd been waiting for this sign

107

since the start of the evening; something in her grew tense, then, she sprang up from the bed and got dressed again tight-lipped, underwear T-shirt, what's up? he asked, lifting himself on to one elbow, frowning – but he knew what was up, don't play dumb she should have said but she just murmured nothing, nothing, nothing's up, while her face grew veiled with bitterness – then he too pulled on his clothes and joined her in the kitchen, where everything went downhill.

Today, in the silence of the empty apartment, leaning over the beginnings of the three-dimensional labyrinth she's building inside a Plexiglas case, she thinks back to it again, how had she slipped so easily into that awful role, the role of the woman who stays behind while the man goes out and enjoys the world, that conjugal pose, that adult thing, that old-people thing, when she is only eighteen; how had she been able to slide to that point, insisting, stay, stay with me, by turns loving and violent, in intonations that weren't her own but those of a fragile and passionate actress, a cliché, reminding him that she had the house to herself this weekend, her parents weren't coming back until Sunday night and they could be together, for a long time, but Simon dug his heels in, it's surfing, that's what it's like, you always decide at the last minute, that's how it is with surf sessions, he too playing the man, and they got stuck, barefoot on the tiles, eyes hard and skin marbled; he tried to take her in his arms, a sudden rush, his hands touching her slim waist beneath the tank top, her hip bones a little pointed, but she had made that brutal gesture, pushing him away, fine, go, don't let me hold you back, and so he left, alright, I'm going, even slammed the door behind him, after saying, with a final look, I'll call you tomorrow, had blown her a kiss on the doorstep.

She's been working on her labyrinth regularly since the new year – all the Grade 12 students taking a visual arts elective are required to present a personal project at the end of the year. She began by building the volume of Plexiglas, one cubic metre, two panes of which would only be placed once it was finished – she had studied samples of material for a long time before choosing – and now she was building the interior. Diagrams at various scales are tacked above her desk, she studies them, moving closer to the wall, and then she places a sheet of white foam board on the work table, prepares the pencils, two metal rulers, clean erasers, a pencil sharpener, and a hot glue gun, goes to wash her hands in the washroom before pulling on a pair of transparent plastic gloves given to her by the hairdresser down the street – they were tucked away in the colourist's cart under trays of dye, between the rollers, multicoloured clips and little sponges.

She begins to notch the white board, using the paper cutter to slice sections that she numbers, following the template she traced to the millimetre which should, once the maquette is done, display a rhizomic starring, complex interlacings where each path crosses another, where there is no entrance, no exit, no centre, but an infinity of paths, connections, branchings, vanishing points, and perspectives. So absorbed in her work that she starts to hear a light hum, as though the silence were vibrating, saturated and enclosing her in a jewel case, placing her in the centre of the world – she loves to draw, mould, cut, glue, sew, has always loved this, her mother and father often bring up the collage menus that she made before she even knew how to read, those little papers she tore up and assembled all day, those mosaics of material sewn with thick strands of yarn, those puzzles, those mobiles that grew more and more sophisticated and that she balanced with

Plasticine, and as they think back on these things, they conjure up the creative child she was, meticulous, passionate, an amazing little girl.

The first time she presented the transparent case to Simon, showing him her project, he asked, perplexed: is it a map of the brain? She looked at him, surprised, and answered, sure of herself, speaking fast: in a way, yeah, it is, it's full of memory, coincidences, questions, it's a space of chance and encounters. She didn't know how to tell him to what extent she experienced all this, each work session causing a kind of detaching that took her far, far away, from her hands, at least, as they moved beneath her eyes; her thoughts escaped as the strips of cardboard piled up on the table and then found a place in the case, glued to the structure with repetitive movements – the pressure of the index on the pistol trigger dosing exactly the right amount of this white hot substance whose odour slowly got her high – drifting slowly toward the lines of the labyrinth, into a mental zone where the hyper-precision of memory mixed with spirals of desire, the great reverie, and always coming back to Simon at the end of the path, coming upon the outline of his tattoo, the lines and dots, the fine scrolls calligraphied in green ink, inevitably ending by meeting him at the whim of an image, because she was in love.

The day stretches out in Juliette's room and little by little the white labyrinth opens a passage to that September day, that first day, the matter of the air slowly taking form once they were finally walking side by side, as though invisible particles were coming together around them under the effect of a sudden acceleration, their bodies sending a signal to each other once they'd passed the high school gates, in the aphonic, archaic language that was already the language of desire; and then, letting her girlfriends go on ahead, she slowed so she would be alone on the pavement when Simon came to fall into step with her, making him out in her mental rear-view mirror, standing up on his bike, right foot on the left pedal, then gliding to earth to escort her, one hand on the handlebars pushing the bike, all this just to talk to her, all this just so they could talk to each other, do you live far from here? I live up on the hill, and you? Close by, just around the corner; the light is wildly clear after rain showers and the pavement is scattered with yellow leaves shaken from the trees, Simon sneaks a sidelong glance, Juliette's skin is so close, fine-grained beneath the blush, her skin is alive, her hair is alive, her mouth is alive as is the lobe of her ear pierced with some gimcrackery, she's drawn a line of eyeliner beneath her lashes, a fawn, do you know Francois Villon, the *Ballade des pendus*? he shakes his head, don't think so, on this day she's wearing raspberry Chapstick, My brothers who live on after us, Don't harden your hearts against us too, do you know it or not? Yeah, I do, but he doesn't know anything, can barely see, he's blinded, thousands of mirrors have formed in the drops of water that vibrate, they lean their heads toward the ground and slalom between puddles, the bike clinking in unison with the rest, each word and each gesture weighted with audacity and reserve like two sides of the same coin, it's the blooming, they are contained within the light of a glass roof, they walk along the avenue like princes, all stirred up but going as slowly as possible, pianissimo, pianissimo, pianissimo, allargando, engulfed in the amazement that they are for each other, their delicateness is incredible, almost molecular, and the thing circling between them pulses a whirling tempo, so that by the time they're at the bottom of the funicular they're short of breath, blood beating in their temporal veins and hands moist, because everything is on the verge of disintegrating now, and at the moment when the bell signals the train's departure, she kisses him on the mouth, an ultrafast kiss, a fluttering of lids, and whoosh, she leaps into the train car, where she turns around and glues her face to the window, forehead suctioned to the grubby glass, he sees her smile and kiss the inside, crush her lips against it, eyes closed, hands flat on the glass, purplish blue lines clearly coding her palms, then she turns around while he stays frozen there, heart impossibly dilated, what just happened?, the funicular starts up and tackles the slope, wheezy, stubborn, and Simon decides to do the same thing only with more grace, puts his bike in gear and begins the ascent, the long loop of the turn makes his path longer but he's pedalling at top speed, pressed low over the bars like a cyclist in a race, his knapsack making a hump on his back, and all at once the sky grows dark, the shadows on the ground disappear, rain again, a maritime rain, heavy, in just a few minutes the pavement streams and the road slides while Simon changes gears and stands up like a dancer, gibbous, blinded by liquid beads suspended along his brow, but so happy in that moment that he could have turned his head up to the sky, opened his mouth and drunk everything that flowed from up there, the muscles in his thighs and calves straining, his forearms aching, he spits, breathes, but finds enough impetus within him to draw the right arc in the final turn at such a perfect angle that he gains speed, reaches the plateau freewheeling, ploughs into the funicular station while the machine's cars brake in a strident screeching, skids in front of the doors, soaking, dripping, gets off his bike and bends forward, hands on his knees, head toward the ground, drool on his lips, locks of hair stuck to the perimeter of his face like a young field marshal, he leans his bike against a bench and catches his breath, undoes his coat, the first buttons of his shirt, the rhythm of his heart slows gradually beneath the tattoo that peeks out, his is the heart of a swimmer in the high seas, the heart of an athlete that, at rest, can lower to under forty beats per minute, bradycardia of an extraterrestrial, but as soon as Juliette passes through the turnstile it all speeds up again, a wave, a surge, hands in his pockets and head tucked between his shoulders, he walks straight toward her, she smiles, takes off her raincoat and holds it up in the air at arm's length, it's an awning, an umbrella, a bed canopy, a photovoltaic panel capable of capturing all the colours in the rainbow, and once they're face to face, she stands up on tiptoe to cover him, and herself with him, both of them contained within this sweetish smell of plastic, and their faces glowing beneath the waxy material, their lashes are navy-blue, their lips purple, their mouths deep and their tongues of an infinite curiosity, they're under the tarp as though under a shelter where everything resonates, the grain pouring down outside forms the sound tableau where breath and hisses of saliva are grafted together, they're under the tarp as though beneath the surface of the world, immersed in a moist clammy space where toads croak, where snails crawl, where a humus of magnolia, browned leaves, linden seeds, and pine needles swells, where balls of chewing gum fester alongside cigarette butts drenched with rain, they're there as though beneath a stained-glass window that resembles daytime on earth, and the kiss goes on and on.

Juliette lifts her head, out of breath, the light has faded, she turns on the lamp and shivers: before her, the labyrinth has grown. She casts a glance at her watch, nearly 5.00 p.m. Simon will be calling soon.

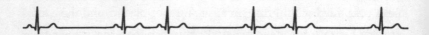

OUTSIDE, THE UNYIELDING SKY BLINDS THEM, LIVID, SHADES of dirty milk, and they lower their heads, rivet their eyes to the tips of their shoes, and walk side by side all the way to the car, hands in their pockets, and noses, mouths and chins buried inside scarves, inside collars. Glacial car, Sean takes the wheel and they slowly manoeuvre out of the parking lot – how many times today through this god-damned gate? They head for the side streets, don't want to be far from the hospital, just want to escape the world, pass below the waterline of this unthinkable day, disappear into an indeterminate, fibrous space, into a diaphanous infrageography that resembles their devastation.

The city stretches, reclines, the last neighbourhoods fray its contour, the pavements wander off, there are no more wooden gates, just high metal fences, a few warehouses and the residue of old urban settlements blackened beneath the rings of highway interchanges, then the shapes of the earth's relief steer their way, guide their drift like lines of force, they drive along the road at the foot of the cliffs, beside the slope crammed with caverns where lone vagabonds hang out, or gangs of kids – dope and spray paint; they pass shacks huddled at the bottom of the slope, the Gonfreville–l'Orcher refinery, finally turn off towards the river, as though compelled by the sudden gap in space, and now the estuary.

They drive another two or three kilometres and then it's the end of the pavement so they cut the motor: it's empty around them, shut down, a space somewhere between an industrial zone and a grazing field, and it's hard to understand why they stop here, beneath a sky wrinkled with thick, dense smoke that twirls above the chimneys of the refinery and dilates into mournful trails, distilling dust and carbon monoxide, an apocalyptic sky. They've barely parked on the roadside when Sean pulls out his pack of Marlboros and starts to smoke without even opening his window. I thought you quit, Marianne gently reaches for his cigarette and takes a drag – she smokes in a very particular way, palm against her mouth, fingers tight and cigarette wedged at the metacarpal joint – lets out the smoke without inhaling, then puts it back between Sean's fingers as he murmurs no, don't want to. She stirs in her seat: are you still the only guy who brushes his teeth with a smoke in his mouth? – summer 1992, a bivouac in the desert near Santa Fe, tie-dyed dawn, somewhere between coral-red and pink monkey palm, a bluish fire, a slice of bacon sizzling in a pan, coffee in white tin mugs, fear of scorpions crouching in the cold shadow of stones, the Rio Bravo song, "My Rifle, My Pony, and Me", sung together, and Sean, the end of a toothbrush smeared with toothpaste propped in a corner of his mouth, a first Marlboro lit at the other end of his smile – he nods his head: yes – the Canadian tent streamed with dew, Marianne was naked under her fringed poncho, hair down to her waist, and was reading, in an exaggeratedly oratorical voice, a collection of poems by Richard Brautigan, found at the back of the Greyhound bus that had dropped them off in Taos.

*

I shouldn't have built him that board. Sean takes the time to crush his smoke in the ashtray and then abruptly slams his head against the steering wheel, bang, his forehead bounces violently back from the hard rubber, Sean! Marianne cries, startled, but he keeps going, speeds up, hitting his head repeatedly, always the same spot on his forehead, bang, bang, bang, stop, stop it right now, Marianne grabs his shoulder to still him, to hold him, but he elbows her away, pushing her so hard her right side hits the door, and while she's shifting back in her seat, he seizes the wheel with his teeth, bites the rubber, lets out a deafening howl, a wild and dark cry, something unbearable, a cry she doesn't want to hear, anything but that, she wants him to stop – she grabs him by the nape, burrows her fingers deep beneath his mane of hair, into the skin of his scalp, she grits her teeth but shouts loudly: stop it right now! And pulls him backwards until his jaw releases the wheel, until his back hits the seat, until his head knocks and then settles against the headrest, eyes closed, space between his two eyes red and burning from the impact, until the cry becomes lamentation, at which point she lets go, trembling, murmurs you shouldn't do that, shouldn't hurt yourself, look at your hand already, she lowers her head, his fingers grip his knees like pliers: Sean, I don't want us to go crazy – and at that very moment, it's possible that it's herself she's talking to, measuring the madness growing in her, in them, madness as though that were the only possible form of thought, the only rational outcome in this unfathomable nightmare.

They sink back together, huddle inside the car, but what seems to be a return to calm is only an illusion, because Sean's howl drills into Marianne's ear, and she suddenly thinks about what this Sunday could have been without the accident, without the exhaustion, without surfing, without this fucking passion for surfing, and at the end of this rope of causality reeled in with a weak hand there's Sean, yes, Sean, that's it, him, he's the one who encouraged this enthusiasm, caused it to come into being and nourished it, canoes, the Maori, tattoos, wooden boards, the ocean, migration to new worlds, affinity with nature, this whole mythical hodgepodge that had fascinated her little boy, this whole fantasy world in cinemascope where he had grown up – she gritted her teeth, would have liked to beat this man beside her, this man who moaned – it was the skiff delivery that they used to do together, she thinks back on it, she and Lou, "just the girls", staying home, put aside, they never missed a *Nuit de la glisse* film, and later Simon had started taking risks, going out more and more often in water that was both too cold and too stormy, and his father never said anything, because he was a laconic and solitary father, an enigmatic father, who had isolated himself to the point that she said to him one night you have to go, I don't want to live with you anymore, not like this, a man she loved still but damn it; yes, surfing, what madness, what dangerous madness, and she, Marianne, how had she let this addiction to strong sensation thrive inside her own house, let her son fall into this spiral of vertigo, the spiral of the tube, that stupid thing, yes, she too had done nothing, hadn't known what to say when her son began living at the whim of the weather, dropping everything when a swell was forecast, homework and all the rest, sometimes getting up at five in the morning to chase a wave a hundred kilometres away, she hadn't done anything, she was in love with Sean and probably fascinated too by this miserable fantasy, the man who builds boats and fires in the snow, knows the names of all the stars and every constellation in the sky, whistles complex melodies, amazed that her son could live so intensely, proud that he was different, and so, they had done nothing, they hadn't known how to protect their child.

*

The condensation that's been forming on the windows starts to drip as Marianne says: the surfboard is the most beautiful thing you ever gave him. He exhales, I don't know, and they are silent. The most beautiful parts were the gestures of making it, what they had shifted in him, the use of foams and resins instead of the supple wood sent to build canoes. In early December he had gone to Les Landes to get sheets of polystyrene from a shaper on the coast – a guy in his fifties with the body of a fakir, forehead girded with a red apache scarf, a grey beard and ponytail, Tahitian Bermudas, a polar fleece and neon flip-flops; a rehashed character then, a man of few words who didn't make eye contact, surfed whenever a session was possible, the luminescent screen of a wireless weather station continually delivering forecasts of wind and the swell – Sean had thought carefully before choosing these materials, unfamiliar to him, had studied their density, their resistance, had opted for extruded polystyrene foam rather than polyurethane, had chosen epoxy resin rather than polyester resin even though the latter was cheaper, had observed the shaper's work for a long time, the speed of the planer and the touch of the sander, had loaded everything up on his truck and sped along the night highway, mulling over the building of the board, mentally tracing its shape, obsessing over its solidity; he had worked in secret.

They get out to walk, come outside says Marianne, already opening her door. They leave the car on the roadside beside a thicket of blackberry bushes that cross their spiny arcs into the ground, and cut through the field, passing beneath the barbed wire fence one after the other – her, then him, one foot, then the other, back flat, each holding the wire up over the other's head, below the belly, watch your hair, your nose, your eyes, careful of your coat.

Wintery bocage. The ground is a cold soup that splat-splats beneath the soles of their shoes, the grass is brittle and the cowpats, hardened by frost, form black slabs here and there, the poplars jut their talons into the sky, and there are crows in the copses, big as hens – all this is so huge, thinks Marianne, it's too much, it's going to kill us.

The river finally comes into view, wild breadth of sky, they're surprised, short of breath, feet soaking wet, but they walk toward the bank, come right to the edge as though magnetised, don't stop until the field begins to slowly pour into the water, dark here, congested with soft branches, decomposing stumps, bodies of insects killed and rotted by the winter, a briny mire, completely still, the pond from a fable, above which the estuary is slow, matte, pale as sage, the fold of a shroud; crossing it seems possible but dangerous, not a single wooden pontoon to suggest the dream, not a single boat anchored there to brave the threat, nor a kid with pockets full of flat stones to draw that leaping light wake on the surface of the water and make them dance, those water spirits that populate the surface; the two of them are trapped there, before the hostile waters, digging their hands into their pockets and their feet into the mud, they face the river, burrow their chins into their collars – what are we doing here? thinks Marianne who wishes she could scream but her wide open mouth lets out not a single sound, nothing, pure nightmare – and then, this boat with a dark hull that drifts in far off to the left, the only visible craft upstream and downstream on the watercourse, a solitary boat that indicates only the absence of all the others.

*

I don't want them to open his body, to skin him, I don't want them to empty him out – chromatic purity of Sean's voice, white – the cold sharpens it like the ash against the blade. Marianne puts her left hand into the right-hand pocket of Sean's parka, her index and middle finger reach the dark crease of his fist, open it, slide inside, widening the passage, tunnelling enough space for her ring finger and little finger to enter in turn, all this without Sean turning his head, the hum of the freighter comes nearer on the left and the colour of the hull becomes clear, an oily red, the exact colour of dried blood, it's a boat loaded with grain, headed downriver, headed for the mouth of the river, headed for the sea, while everything widens, waters and consciousnesses, everything converges toward the open, toward the unformed and the infinity of loss, it's suddenly enormous, out of scale and so close it feels as if they could touch it with an outstretched finger, it passes, casting its cold shadow over them, everything shudders, everything's stirred up and thrown into turmoil, Marianne and Sean follow it with their eyes, long hull, a hundred and eighty metres, thirty thousand tonnes at least, it files past, red curtain sliding progressively towards reality – and what they're thinking in that moment, I couldn't say, they're probably thinking of Simon, where he was before he was born, where he is now; or maybe they're not thinking of anything at all, seeing only this vision of the world that's gradually revealed, appearing anew, tangible, absolutely enigmatic – and the prow that cleaves the water affirms the searing present of their pain.

The boat's wake churns and subsides, smooths, the freighter moves farther away, carrying with it the noise and movement, the river returns to its initial texture, and the estuary is set aflame, a radiance. Marianne and Sean have turned toward each other, are holding hands, arms held out from their bodies, and they've caressed each other with their faces – nothing more tender than this sanding, nothing more gentle than the bony ridges of the facial massif that run beneath the skin – in the end they hold each other up, forehead to forehead, and Marianne's words make an imprint in the static air.

They won't hurt him, they won't hurt him at all. Her voice is caught in a textile filter, and Sean lets go of her hands to take her in his arms, her sobs prolong the breathing of nature, okay, he says, it's time for us to go back.

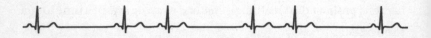

– HE'LL BE A DONOR.

Sean is the one to make this statement and Thomas Remige gets up from his chair abruptly, shaky, red, thorax expanding with an influx of heat as though his blood were speeding up, and walks straight toward them. Thank you. Marianne and Sean lower their eyes, planted like stakes in the office doorway, wordless, their shoes mark the floor, leave sludge and black grass, they themselves are overwhelmed by what they've just done, by what they've just announced – "donor", "donor", "don-ate", "aban-don", the words clang together in the hollow of their eardrums, bore in one after the other. The phone rings, it's Revol, Thomas tells him quickly that it's a go, three quick words in a cryptic language that Sean and Marianne don't catch, acronyms and the speed of elocution intended to scramble comprehension, and soon they leave the coordinator's office to go back to the room where they had their meeting. Revol is there waiting for them – there are four of them at present and they slip back into the dialogue immediately because Marianne whispers, still standing: now, what happens now?

*

It's five-thirty. The window is open as though the atmosphere in the room needed to be refreshed, made new, the preceding dialogue having exhausted it, spoiled it – breath, tears, sweat. Outside: a strip of lawn at the base of the wall, a paved path, and between the two, a hedge as tall as a man. Thomas Remige and Pierre Revol take their places in the vermilion chairs while Marianne and Sean return to the apple-green couch, and their anguish is palpable – still this widening of the eyes that creases the forehead and augments the white around the iris, still these half-open lips, ready to scream, and the whole body's attention made brittle by the wait, by fear. They're not cold, not yet.

We're going to begin an evaluation of all organs, and transmit this information to the doctor at the Agency of Biomedicine who will recommend the harvesting of one or several of them. Then we'll schedule the procedure itself in the operating room. Your child's body will be returned to you tomorrow morning. These words are Revol's, and he joins a gesture of his hand to the ledge of each sentence, tracing the steps of the next sequence in the air. There's a lot of information in these sentences, which nevertheless leave a stark gap in the middle, an opaque zone that catalyzes their fear: the procedure itself.

Sean speaks up suddenly: what are they going to do to him, exactly? He said "exactly" – didn't emit that strangled stammering but stretched out his question, brave in this moment, a soldier advancing under heavy fire, breast offered to the machine gun, while Marianne clenches her teeth on the sleeve of her coat. What will happen tonight within the enclave of the operating room, the idea they have of it, this parcelling out of Simon's body, this dispersion – it horrifies them but they still want to know. Remige takes a deep breath before replying: they make an incision, they harvest, and they close it up again.

Simple verbs, action verbs, atonal information to counteract the drama linked to the sanctity of the body, to the transgression of opening it.

Are you the one who will operate? Sean lifts his forehead – always this impression that he's going to charge, from below, like a boxer. In sync, Revol and Remige discern the part of the question that comes from a continent of archaic terror: to be pronounced dead, straight from the mouths of doctors, when one is in fact alive – we'll remember that Revol keeps a copy of the thriller *Moonlight Becomes You* by Mary Higgins Clark in his office, a book that refers to a common funerary practice in England: they would put a ring on the finger of the person being buried, a ring tied to a cord that would cause a bell to sound on the surface if the person ever woke up underground; and the "custom-made" definition of the criteria of death, established in order to allow for retrieval, gets mixed in with this immemorial fear. The nurse turns to face Sean, inscribes a solemn sign in the air with his thumb and index finger: the doctors who pronounce a patient's death never participate in the process of organ retrieval, never; plus – he firms each sound and his voice grows wider, deeper – there's always a double procedure, two doctors follow the same protocol and two separate signatures are required on the written record that attests to a death – squelching the scenario of the criminal doctor who wittingly decrees the death of his patient in order to ransack him, crushing the rumours that link medical mafia to the international trafficking of organs, invisible dispensaries squeezed into the stringy suburbs of Pristina, Dacca or Mumbai, and discreet clinics pro-tected by video cameras and shaded beneath palm trees in the upscale neighbourhoods of Western metropolises. Remige concludes, gently: the surgeons who will harvest are from hospitals where there are patients waiting for transplants.

*

Stream of silence, then Marianne's voice again, muffled, as though coming from inside a membranous pouch: but then who will be with Simon? – stress on "who", naked as a stone. I will, Thomas replies, I'm there, I'm there for the whole process. Marianne slowly pours her gaze into his – transparency of crushed glass – so you'll tell them about his eyes, that we don't want, you'll tell them. Thomas nods, I will tell them, yes. He gets up, but Sean and Marianne wait, unmoving, a force weighs on their shoulders and grinds them into the ground, this lasts for a moment, and then Marianne continues: we don't know who will get Simon's heart, right, it's anonymous, we'll never know, right? And Thomas agrees with these affirmations that question, these questions that affirm, he understands the oscillation, but clarifies: you can be informed of the sex and the age of the recipient, yes, but not their identity; however, if you wish, you can be kept informed about the transplant. Then he unfurls a little further: the heart, if it ends up being transplanted, will be given to a patient according to medical and compatibility criteria that have nothing to do with gender, but, given Simon's age, his organs are likely to go to children. Sean and Marianne listen and then confer in low voices. Sean says: we'd like to go back to see Simon now.

Revol gets up, he's needed elsewhere in the department, Thomas accompanies Marianne and Sean to the doorway of the room, they walk in silence, I'll leave you now with Simon, I'll meet you later.

Evening has darkened the room and the silence, it seems, is even thicker than before. They approach the bed with its unmoving folds. They must have thought that Simon's appearance would have altered after the announcement of his death, or that at least something in his aspect would have changed since the last time – the colour of his skin, the texture, glow, or temperature. But no, nothing. Simon is there, unchanged, the micro-movements of his body still lift the sheet lightly, so that what they've gone through doesn't correspond to anything, doesn't find any confirmation, and this is such a violent blow that their thinking comes unhinged, they flail and stammer, a rodeo, speak to Simon as though he could hear them, talk about him as though he couldn't hear them anymore, seem to struggle to remain in language while sentences disarticulate, words knock together, become fragmented and short-circuit, while caresses collide, become breaths; sounds and signs soon whittled down to a continuous hum inside ribcages, an imperceptible vibration as though they are henceforth expelled from all language, and their actions find neither time nor place to fit into, and then, lost in the crevasses of reality, lost in its flaws, themselves flawed, broken, disunited, Sean and Marianne find the strength to heave themselves on to the bed to be closer to the body of their child, Marianne stretching out along the railing at the edge, hair falling into the void while Sean, one thigh on the mattress, leans over and rests his head on Simon's chest, his mouth right over the tattoo, and his parents close their eyes together and are quiet, as though they, too, are sleeping; night has fallen and they're in the dark.

Two floors down, Thomas Remige is glad of this moment alone when he can concentrate, review the process, and call the Agency of Biomedicine: we're moving on to an in-depth assessment of the organs – the woman at the other end of the line is a pioneer of the organisation, Thomas recognises her deep, raspy voice, pictures her in the middle of a classroom with tables set in a U-shape, the big amber-coloured plastic links in her glasses chain concealing her face – then he sits down in front of the computer, and, following a labyrinthine path that requires him to enter several identification numbers and encrypted passwords, he opens a program and creates a new document where he carefully inputs all the data for Simon Limbeau's body: it's the Cristal file, archive and dialoguing tool that is currently being developed with the Agency of Biomedicine to ensure the traceability of the graft and the anonymity of the donor. He lifts his head: a bird hops on the windowsill outside, the same one as always, its eyes are fixed and round.

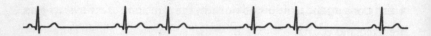

THE DAY THOMAS ACQUIRED THE GOLDFINCH, THE HEAT MADE Algiers disappear beneath a cloud of steam, and inside his apartment with the indigo blinds, Hocine was fanning himself, legs bare under a striped djellaba, stretched out on a sofa.

The stairwell was painted blue, it smelled of cardamom and concrete. Ousmane and Thomas climbed three flights in the dimness, the frosted glass slabs on the roof filtering a yellow quivering light that struggled to reach the main floor. Reunion of cousins – a strong embrace and then a rapid conversation in Arabic punctuated by the clicking of pistachios between teeth – Thomas is left out. He doesn't recognise Ousmane's face that distorts differently when he speaks his language – jaw retracting, gums appearing, eyes rolling and sounds arising from the back of his throat, issued from a complicated zone far behind the tonsils, new vowels held back and then clacked against the palate: he's almost a different person, almost a stranger, and Thomas is unsettled. The visit takes a completely different turn when Ousmane announces, in French, the reason for their visit: my friend would like to hear the goldfinches. Ah, Hocine turns to Thomas, and maybe adopt one? he asks, winking at him, laying it on thick. Maybe. Thomas smiles.

Having arrived the day before and crossed the Mediterranean for the first time, the young man is captivated by the Bay of Algiers, arced in a curve of perfection, and by the city behind that lays itself out in tiers, the whites and blues, youth in great numbers, the smell of mist-sprayed pavements, the dragon trees interlinking their branches in the botanical gardens, arches from a *fantastique* literary tale. An unvoluptuous, stripped-down beauty. He's intoxicated. New sensations grasp and discombobulate him, a mix of sensorial thrill and the hyperconsciousness of everything that surrounds him: life is here, no filter, and he is here too. The bills rolled inside the little handkerchief form a bump in his pocket – he pats it in a sign of euphoric excitement.

Hocine goes out on to the balcony, pushes open the shutters and leans into the street, claps his hands, tosses out orders, Ousmane protests in Arabic, seems to be saying, no, please, don't trouble yourself, pleading, but here they are sending up soups and kebabs, plates of grain light as mousse, orange salad with mint, and honey cakes. After the meal, Hocine places the cages on the ceramic tiles that line the ground, using their patterns as markers to align them perfectly. The birds are tiny – twelve to thirteen centimetres – and all throat, the abdomen disproportionate, the feathers unspectacular, matchstick claws, and all with the same fixed eyes. They're perched on little wooden trapezes that swing lightly. Thomas and Ousmane crouch a few feet from the cages while Hocine curls up on an ottoman at the back of the room. He lets out a cry comparable to a yodel and the recital begins: the birds sing, one by one, and then together – a canon. The two boys don't dare look at each other, don't dare touch.

And yet, it was said everywhere that goldfinches were disappearing. The ones from the Bainem forest, the ones from Kadous and from

Dély Ibrahim, the ones from Souk Ahras. There were none left. Unchecked hunting threatened the extinction of populations that were once so dense. In the doorways of rooms in the Casbah, hanging cages creaked, empty, while those of the merchants were gradually decorated with canaries and budgies, but not a single goldfinch, unless it was tucked away in the darkness at the back of the shop, guarded like a treasure, the bird's value increasing with its rarity – the law of capitalism. You might be able to buy them still on Friday evenings in El Harrach, to the east of the city, but everyone knew that the specimens on display there, like those of the Bab El Oued market, had never flown along the Algerian hillsides, never nested in the branches of pines and cork oaks that grew there, and had not been captured in a traditional way, with birdlime, where females that didn't sing would be immediately released to ensure reproduction: they didn't have the gift. No, these ones came from the Moroccan border, from the Maghnia region where they were hunted in the thousands, the ornithological net making a clean sweep, no distinction between males and females, and then were brought to the capital via channels manned by guys not yet even twenty who dickered in the trade, unemployed kids who'd abandoned their moribund jobs to dabble in this trafficking, sure their revenues would be juicier, guys who knew nothing about birds – and most of the specimens, throttled in nets, died of stress during the transport.

Hocine raised expensive birds behind the Square of Three Clocks, Algerian goldfinches, real ones. He always had at least a dozen in his possession and had never had any other job; his expert status was known throughout Bab El Oued and beyond. Recognised each species, characteristics and metabolism, could tell the provenance of each bird by ear, even the name of its native forest; people came from far and wide to call upon his services, to authenticate, estimate, uncover swindles – Moroccan specimens sold as Algerian, sometimes for ten times more, females sold as males. Hocine didn't deal with the networks, he did his hunting himself, alone, with birdlime; he would leave on foot for several days, claiming to have "his" spots in the valleys of Bejaia and Collo, and when he returned would spend the better part of his time cherishing his catches. Since the superiority of one goldfinch over another was measured by the beauty of its song, he worked at teaching them airs – the birds from Souk Ahras had a reputation for being able to memorise a great quantity – using an old tape player that broadcast its melody in the mornings, on repeat, never subscribing to the methods of younger breeders – covering the cages, making two slits, inserting MP3 earphones that played all night. But even more than musicality, what the goldfinch delivered was emotion, and this mostly around geography: its song made a territory materialise. Valley, city, mountain, wood, hill, stream. It made a landscape appear, made you feel a topography, touch a certain ground and climate. A piece of the planetary puzzle took shape in its beak, and, like the sisters in the fairy tale who spit out toads or diamonds, like the crow in the fable that shelled out cheese, the goldfinch coughed up a solid entity, one that was aromatic, tactile, and full of colour. Hocine's eleven birds, a variety, thus delivered the sonorous cartography of an entire, vast region.

His clients, businessmen in ties sporting gold-rimmed sunglasses and usually squeezed into light grey or beige suits, would turn up at his place in the middle of the afternoon like jonesing addicts. The birds sang, the buyers remembered running in sandals through pine needles, remembered armfuls of cyclamen and saffron milk caps, undid a few buttons, drank lemonade and, since the song determined the value of one bird over another, the prices ranged. Hocine did well. One day, the young heir of an oil company traded his car, a 205 GTI, for the last goldfinch from Baïnem that he ever held in his hands, a coup that established the breeder as a legend – and stoic, too: the bird was well worth that much, more mythic than the djinn of fairy tales or the genie in the magic lamp – this was not just a bird, it was an endangered forest and the sea that borders it, and all that inhabits it, the part for the whole, Creation itself – this was childhood.

After the concert, the palavering began. Which one do you like? Hocine asked Thomas – he brought his face very close. Ousmane watched his friend, amused, thoroughly enjoying the situation. Which one do you like, tell me, don't be afraid, I like them all! Thomas pointed to a cage – inside, the creature stopped swinging. Hocine cast a glance at Ousmane and nodded his head. They exchanged a few words in Arabic.

Ousmane started to laugh. Thomas thought he was being played, he took a step back, behind the cages. The silence dilated, Thomas's hand slid inside his pocket, his fingers fondled the handkerchief. He paced conspicuously, not daring to say let's go. Hocine announced the price for the bird he had pointed out. Ousmane said softly, it's a bird from Collo, ash, elm, eucalyptus, he's young, you'll be able to raise him, teach him, it's a bird from my village. Thomas, suddenly spellbound, stroked the creature's back through the bars of the cage, thought for a long moment, then unrolled the roll of bills – I hope you got your commission, he said to Ousmane as they went back down the stairs.

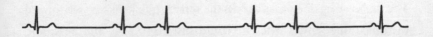

SEAN AND MARIANNE LEAVE THE ROOM. THOMAS IS THERE, JUST
outside, waiting for them. They open their mouths but remain mute,
seem as if they want to speak, concerted words, Thomas engages
them, I'm listening, that's what I'm here for, and Sean articulates their
request with difficulty: Simon's heart, at the moment when, tell
Simon, when you stop his heart, I, for, you have to tell him, we're
there, with him, that we're thinking of him, our love, and Marianne
continues: and Lou, and Juliette too, and Grammy; then Sean again:
the sound of the sea, so he can hear it, he holds out a pair of earphones and an MP3 player to Thomas, track seven, it's ready, it's so he
can hear the sea – strange loops in their brains – and Thomas agrees
to carry out these rites, in their name, it will be done.

They're about to leave, but Marianne turns around one last time
toward the bed and what freezes her in place then is the solitude that
emanates from Simon, from now on as alone as an object, as though
he had been unballasted of his human aspect, as though he were no
longer linked to a community, joined to a network of intentions and
emotions, but rather erred in another space, transformed into something absolute; Simon is dead, she says these words to herself for the
first time, suddenly horrified, looks for Sean but can't see him, rushes

into the corridor, finds him prostrate slumped against the wall, he too irradiated by Simon's solitude, he, too, certain now of his death. She crouches in front of him, tries to lift his head by cupping her hands beneath his chin, come, come on, let's leave this place – what she would like to say is: it's over, come, Simon doesn't exist anymore.

The mobile rings, Thomas checks the screen, quickens his step toward his office, suddenly wishes he could just run there, and Sean and Marianne who are walking beside him catch this acceleration, understand instinctively that they have to make room, and feel suddenly cold – these same overheated corridors that dried out their skin and left their mouths thirsting have become icy alleyways where they do up their coats, turn up their collars. Simon's body will be made to disappear, whisked away to a secret place with controlled access, the O.R., the operating theatre, his body will be opened, stripped of its organs, closed again, sewn up, and for a lapse of time – the length of one night – the course of events is completely beyond their control.

The situation suddenly topples into another, different urgency, pressure streams through their movements, their gestures, no longer clanging in their consciousness – now it flows elsewhere, into the office of the organ donation specialist where Thomas Remige is already talking with the doctor from the Agency of Biomedicine, into the movements of the stretcher bearers who carry the body of their son, flows into the eyes that analyse images on screens, flows far away, into other hospitals and other departments, on to other beds that are just as white, into other houses that are just as grief-stricken, and from now on they don't know quite what to do anymore, they're lost; of course they could stay here in the department, sit down before worn newspapers, before dog-eared magazines with dirty edges, wait until six o'clock when the second electroencephalogram will be finished, the one that will legally certify Simon's death, or go downstairs to get a coffee from the vending machine, they can do what they like, but they are gently told that preparing for the retrieval of multiple organs takes several hours, they should be aware, and then the operation itself takes time, it doesn't happen quickly, so they are encouraged to go home, you should probably rest a little, you're going to need your strength, we'll take care of him — and when they pass through the automatic doors of the hospital's large nave, they are alone in the world, and fatigue crashes over them, a tidal wave.

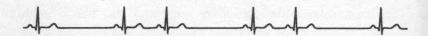

SHE GOT OFF THE R.E.R. AT DAWN, LA PLAINE-STADE DE FRANCE station, and walked in exactly the opposite direction to that which the multitude takes now, the masses disgorged in a continuous flow that gets more and more compact as the kick-off draws near, all amalgamated into a collective fever – pre-game excitement and conjectures, fine-tuning of chants and insults, Delphic oracles. She turned her back on the enormous, naked stadium, indifferent to its massive anchorage, off-the-scale, as absurd and incontestable as a flying saucer landed in the night; sped up her step through the short tunnel that passes beneath the tracks and then, in the open air again, walked two hundred metres up Stade-de-France Avenue, past the head offices of service providers, banks, insurance companies and other organisations, their facades smooth, white, metallic, transparent, and once she reached number one, she rummaged in her purse for a long moment, then took her gloves off to search better, and finally dumped everything out on the ground in front of the entrance; she knelt on the freezing pavement beneath the indifferent gaze of the guy inside who was uncapping a yogurt drink with infinite care in order to avoid the least spot on his handsome navy suit, and then, as though by a miracle, her fingers touched the magnetic card at the bottom of a pocket.

136

She picked up all her things and headed into the atrium. I'm on duty, I'm a doctor at the Agency of Biomedicine, she said without looking at him, haughty, strode across the hall, past the desk, where her practised eye fell on the pack of Marlboro Lights lying beside the digital tablet he probably used to watch movies all night, soccer and trash, she thought, irritated, and once she reached the second floor, walked twenty metres down the hallway to the left and pushed upon the door of the National Organ Allocation office.

Marthe Carrare is a short woman, around sixty, olive-skinned and round, auburn hair, voluminous breasts and abdomen stuffed inside a tight camel-coloured cardigan, spherical buttocks bobbing in brown wool trousers, and then a pair of rather skinny legs and tiny feet bulging inside flat loafers; she lives on cheeseburgers and nicotine chewing gum, and at the moment her right ear is red and swollen from pressing various telephone receivers against it all day – professional cell, personal cell, landline – and it would be wise not to pester her with trivialities, it would be wise to remain silent and invisible while she asks Thomas to fill her in on the situation: so, where are we at? He replies: it's going ahead. She's calm: okay, send me his death certificate so I can consult the file, and Thomas's voice can be heard saying: I just faxed it to you, I also filled in the donor's Cristal file.

Marthe hangs up, goes over to the fax machine, forehead furrowed along the vertical above the bridge of her nose, thick-framed glasses with a faux-gold chain, lipstick disappearing into tiny wrinkles, heady perfume and old tobacco vapours trapped beneath her collar, the paper is indeed there – the official report certifying the death of Simon Limbeau at 6.36 p.m. – and now she heads into the adjoining office that holds the organ and tissue donor registry, a highly classified file that only a dozen people are authorised to access, and only once a death is certified by a legal document.

Back in her office, Marthe Carrare lets Thomas know she's received everything, then rivets her eyes to the computer screen, opens the Cristal folder, clicks on the different documents contained within, a file with general information, the medical evaluation of each organ, scans, ultrasounds, and various analyses; she studies the whole thing, right away noting Simon Limbeau's relatively rare blood group (B negative). The file is complete. Marthe pushes Enter and gives him an ID number, this will guarantee the anonymity of the donor: from now on, Simon Limbeau's name will not appear in the exchanges between the agency and the different affiliated hospitals. The protocol for the distribution of organs begins. One liver, two lungs, two kidneys. And a heart.

Night falls. At the end of the street, the stadium is lit up and its oblong ring shape – a bean – traces a greyish halo in the sky that skims the bellies of Sunday night airplanes. It's time now to turn to those who are waiting, scattered across the country and sometimes beyond its borders, people registered on lists according to the organ to be transplanted, and who wake up each morning wondering if their place on the list has shifted, if they've moved up on the sheet of paper, people who can't even conceive of a future and are living constrained lives, stranded by the state of their ailing organ. Imagine having a sword of Damocles poised over your head like that – just think of it.

Their medical files are centralised in the computer that Marthe Carrare uses now, sucking on a nicotine tablet and realising, after a glance at her watch, that she's forgotten to cancel dinner with her daughter and son-in-law, supposed to happen in two hours; she doesn't like going to their place, she articulates it to herself clearly now, I don't like going there, it's so cold – but wouldn't be able to say whether it was the apartment walls daubed with nice casein white paint that make her shiver, or rather the absence of an ashtray and a balcony, meat, mess, or tension; or maybe it's the stools from Mali and the designer chaise longue, the vegetarian soups served in Moorish stoneware, the scented candles (Cut Grass, Wood Fire, Wild Mint), the stylish satisfaction of those who go to bed with the chickens under comforters of Indian velvet, the tender atony distilled throughout their kingdom; or maybe it's the couple that frightens her, this couple that, in less than two years, has swallowed up her only daughter, disintegrated her into a sure, emollient conjugality, a balm after years of solitary nomadism: her spirited, polyglot daughter has become completely unrecognisable.

Marthe Carrare enters all the medical data for Simon Limbeau's heart, lungs, liver and kidneys into a web interface, then launches the search engine to scan the waiting lists for patients fit to receive them – the more complicated organs to match are the liver and kidneys. Once compatible recipients are identified, the feasibility of the transplant combines with geographical reality: the location of organ retrieval and location of transplants trace a high-pressure cartography involving distances to be covered within a strictly limited time – that of the organs' viability – and require them to think logistics, to evaluate kilometres and lengths of time, to locate airports and highways, train stations, pilots and planes, specialised transport and experienced drivers, and so the geographical aspect adds a new parameter to the identification of a handful of patients.

*

The first match between donor and recipient is the blood group – the ABO compatibility. A heart transplant requires a compatible ABO and Rh factor, and since Simon Limbeau is B negative, a first skimming shortens the initial list that contained nearly three hundred patients waiting for a transplant – Marthe Carrare's fingers fly over the keyboard, and you can feel her rushing in search of the recipient, intoxicated, perhaps, at this moment, forgetting everything else. Next she examines the tissue compatibility with the H.L.A. system, equally essential: the H.L.A. code (Human Leucocyte Antigen) is the subject's biological ID, involved in immune defence and, although it's practically impossible to find a donor with an H.L.A. identity that is exactly identical to the recipient's, these codes must be as close as possible for the transplant to have the best chance of success, and in order to lower the risk of a rejection.

Marthe Carrare has entered Simon's age into the computer application, and so the list of paediatric receivers is consulted in priority. Then she checks whether there's a compatible patient on the high-emergency national list, a patient whose life is in danger, who could die from one moment to the next and thus has a priority position on this list – she, too, carefully follows a sophisticated protocol, in which each step is dictated by the previous one and determines the next to come. For the heart, besides the blood-type and immune system compatibility, the physical structure of the organ, its morphology, and its dimensions come into play, the size and weight criteria further whittling down the list of potential recipients – the heart of a tall, strong adult cannot be transplanted into the body of a child, for example, nor the inverse – and the geography parameters for the

140

transplant are determined by an intangible fact: between the moment when the heart is stopped inside the body of the donor and the moment when it begins to beat again inside that of the recipient, the organ can be stored for a maximum of four hours.

The research crystallises and Marthe moves her face toward the screen, her eyes enormous and anamorphosed behind the lenses of her glasses. Abruptly, her fingers – yellowed along the inner edge of the third phalange – stop the mouse: an emergency is identified for the heart – a woman, fifty-one years old, blood group B, five feet, six inches, 143 pounds, a patient at Pitié-Salpêtrière, the teaching hospital in Paris, in Professor Harfang's ward. She takes her time carefully reading and rereading the data onscreen, knows that the call she's about to make will cause a general and marked acceleration at the other end of the line, an influx of electricity in brain synapses, an injection of energy in bodies – in other words: hope.

Hi, this is the Agency of Biomedicine – surfeit of diligence and attention from the department's reception – calls bounce from switchboard to extensions and all the way to the operating room, and then a voice cuts straight through, Harfang here, and Marthe Carrare launches in, fast and direct, Doctor Carrare, Agency of Biomedicine, I have a heart – it's crazy, she says it in these terms, vocal cords with their patina of forty years of cigarettes and nicotine balls batted back and forth against her palatal fossa – I have a heart for a patient in your ward who's waiting for a transplant, a compatible heart. Immediate response – not the least sliver of silence – okay, send me the file. And Carrare concludes: it's done, you have twenty minutes.

Then Marthe Carrare descends a line on the list of recipients onscreen and calls the teaching hospital in Nantes, another cardiac surgical department where the same dialogue plays out concerning a seven-year-old child who has been waiting nearly forty days – Carrare specifies, we are waiting for an answer from the Pitié, then, once again: you have twenty minutes. A third department is also contacted at the Timone hospital in Marseille.

The wait begins, its tempo measured by telephone calls between the doctor in Saint-Denis and the coordinator in Le Havre, in order to synchronise arrangements for the operation, to prepare the O.R. and the operating teams, and to be as informed as possible about the donor's haemodynamic condition – stable for the moment. Marthe Carrare knows Thomas Remige well, has met him several times in training courses organised by the agency, seminars where she gave presentations both as an anaesthetist and as a pioneer of the organisation, and she's glad that he's her spokesperson now, she trusts him, knows he's reliable, technical and courteous, he's someone you can count on, they say, and she probably appreciates him all the more because his focus keeps a lid on his agitation, never letting anything other than level-headed intensity show, and because he disparages the dramatic plains of hysteria even though it would often be so easy to take advantage of the human tragedy that lies just behind all organ transplant procedures – the whole world can call itself lucky to have a guy like him around.

Responses for the liver, the kidneys and the lungs come one after the other following this same procedure – Strasbourg will take the liver (a little six-year-old girl), Lyon the lungs (a seventeen-year-old girl), Rouen the kidneys (a nine-year-old boy) – while over there, in the twists and turns of the stadium, jackets are unzipped sharply, the same way you'd set a plan in action, *zzzzip* – black leather jackets, khaki bombers with orange linings –scarves are pulled over faces like bandits when they attack the stagecoach or students at a protest when the teargas is released, and hundreds of smoke grenades are pulled out by expert hands, smuggled in under sweaters, tucked in the back of waistbands, stuffed inside pants – but how did these objects make it past security? The pins are pulled out of the first ones when the players' buses arrive at Porte de la Chapelle, red smoke, green smoke, white smoke, the clamour intensifies in the bleachers as a long banner is unfolded, "Managers, players, coaches, go home!" – the extremist bleachers flex their muscles, compact, brimming, a block of power and aggression, a hostile mass, and those who are just arriving rush forward, rapt, while the security guards' foreheads grow furrowed with lines and they set off at a gallop, bundled into their suits, jackets unbuttoned and ties flapping against paunches, they yell into walkie-talkies, the north section is getting worked up, we can't let it get out of hand, names of birds burst out, the buses with tinted windows have just turned off the highway, comfortable and fantastically silent vehicles currently driving along V.I.P. routes that enlace the arena, finally stopping before the entrances reserved for players. Marthe gets up, opens the window: silhouettes pass before the building of the agency and rush up the avenue towards the stadium, young people from the neighbourhood who know the territory, she sends a laconic text to her daughter – emergency at the abm, call you tomorrow, Mum – and then taps the box of gum against the balcony railing, digs a finger beneath the dispenser tab, discovers the box is empty, and bites her lip – she knows she's scattered cigarettes all across this office, inventing hiding places she's not sure she'll be able to find again now, but for the moment decides to chew a little longer.

She imagines thousands of people assembled in a circle over there, around a field of such brilliant green you'd think it had been varnished with a brush, each blade of grass illuminated by a substance mixing resin and essence of turpentine or lavender and which, after the evaporation of the solvent, would have formed this solid and transparent film like a silvery sheen, like a coating on new cotton, a waxed sail, and thinks that at the moment of matching Simon Limbeau's living organs, at the moment of sharing them out between ailing bodies, thousands of lungs are inflating together over there, thousands of livers are being inundated with beer, thousands of kidneys are filtering the body's substances in unison, thousands of hearts are pumping in the atmosphere, and suddenly she is struck by the fragmentation of the world, by the absolute discontinuity of reality, humanity pulverised into an infinite divergence of trajectories – an anguished feeling she has felt before, that day in March in 1984, sitting in the 69 bus heading to a clinic in the 19th arrondissement for an abortion, less than six months after the birth of her daughter whom she was raising alone; rain streamed down the windows and she had looked one by one at the faces of the few passengers around her, faces you see in Parisian buses in the middle of the morning, faces with eyes fleeting toward the faraway or riveted to safety instructions listed within a pictogram, fixated on the emergency button, lost inside the pavilion of a human ear, eyes that avoid each other, old women with shopping bags, young mothers with children in carriers, retired folks heading for the city library to read their daily paper, chronically unemployed people in dubious suits and ties, plunged into their newspapers although they can't manage to read a single line, not the tiniest glint of sense springing forth from the page, but they cling to the paper as though to keep their heads above water in a world that has no room for them anymore, where soon they won't have enough to live on, people sometimes sitting less than twenty centimetres away from her, none of whom know what she is about

144

to do, this decision she has made and that, in two hours, will be irreversible, people who are living their lives and with whom she shares nothing, nothing, besides this bus caught in a sudden downpour, these worn-out seats and these sticky plastic handholds suspended from the ceiling like nooses knotted to hang yourself, nothing – each one has a life, each one their own, that's all, and she had felt that her eyes were swimming in tears, had squeezed the metal bar harder so she wouldn't fall, and in that moment she probably felt it: the true experience of solitude.

The first police car sirens are heard around seven-thirty. She closes the window again – the cold – an hour still until kick-off, it will be difficult to keep the fans' excitement under control, all those hearts together is too much, who's playing tonight? Time passes. Marthe Carrare looks at the first folder again, strangely satisfied by how well it matches the donor's file, they won't find a better one, what are they waiting for at the Pitié? In that very second the phone rings, it's Harfang: we'll take it.

Marthe Carrare hangs up and calls Le Havre right away, tells Thomas that a team from the Pitié-Salpêtrière will contact him to coordinate his arrival, the recipient is a patient in Harfang's ward, do you know Harfang? I know the name. She smiles, adds: they have a good team there, they know what they're doing. Thomas checks his watch, says: okay, we'll go ahead with the harvesting, we should be in O.R. in about three hours, we'll be in touch. They hang up. Harfang. Marthe says his name aloud. Harfang. She knows it too. Knew it even before she knew him, this strong name, this strange name that's been running through the corridors of Parisian hospitals for more than a century – so that now people would say it's a Harfang to conclude an exchange that had demonstrated the excellence of a practitioner, and they spoke of the "Harfang dynasty" to describe the family that had produced professors and practitioners by the dozen, Charles-Henris and Louises, Juleses, then Roberts and Bernards, and today Mathieus, Gilleses and Vincents, doctors who had all worked, worked still in public institutions – and as they run the New York marathon in the autumn, ski at Courchevel in winter, or regatta in the Gulf of Morbihan on single-hulled carbon boats in spring and summer, they like to say to themselves, we are servants of the state, thus distinguishing themselves from the greedy medical plebs, when in fact a number of them, among the youngest, went directly from finishing residency to opening private clinics in quiet, leafy neighbourhoods, sometimes going into partnership with other Harfangs in order to cover the whole spectrum of pathologies of the human body and to offer quick checkups to overweight businessmen, guys in a rush who are worried by surfeits of cholesterol, capillary desertification, prostate hassles, and declining libido – among them are five generations of pulmonologists, comfy within this patrilineal filiation that privileges the male primogeniture, every time, when the moment comes to pass on appointments as chair and department head; among them, one girl, Brigitte, who ranked first in residency in Paris in 1952 but left the profession two years later, persuaded that she was in love with one of her father's protégés when really she was just giving in to a surreptitious pressure telling her she should make room, increase the vital space for young males of the clan; and him, Emmanuel Harfang, the surgeon.

Marthe remembers hanging out with a group headed by a pair of Harfang cousins during her residency. One was in paediatric cardiology, the other in gynaecology. They had the "Harfang feather", the same shock of white hair growing in a cowlick in the middle of their foreheads that they pushed back with a flick of the wrist – familial seal and visual marker, the vapour trail of a legend, follow my white plume and the whole impromptu swagger designed to soften women's vigilance; they wore Levi's 501s and Oxford shirts, plaid-lined beige raincoats with the collars turned up, never went out in sneakers, wore Church's even though they disdained tasselled loafers, stood at medium height, knobbly, with pale skin and golden eyes, thin lips, and Adam's apples so protruding that Marthe too would begin to swallow when she saw them slide beneath the skin of their throats; they looked like each other and also like this Emmanuel Harfang who mends and transplants hearts at the Pitié-Salpêtrière, only ten years younger.

This last one descends the stairs of the auditorium exactly as the symposium starts, looking straight ahead, skipping the last step so he might be carried forward by his momentum and reach the desk with an athletic bound, a paper in his hand that he won't read, beginning his talk without even greeting the audience, preferring blunt leads, abrupt openings, a way of getting straight to the point without adhering to etiquette, without weakening his family name, as though each person in the room was supposed to know already who he was – Harfang, son of Harfang, grandson of Harfang – and a way also, no doubt, of perking up an audience that has a tendency to nod off in the early afternoon, a little dulled after those infamous meals in nearby restaurants reserved for the occasion, improvised refectories where carafes of red wine are lined up on paper napkins, always that modest, full-bodied Corbières that goes well with rare meat, and from Harfang's first words, the room emerges from its digestive torpor, each one remembering, as they watch him so slim and athletic up there, that he is the pillar of a top-ranking cycling club, a team that wears the hospital colours in various races, guys able to ride two hundred kilometres on Sunday mornings as long as it fits in with department life, guys ready to get up at the crack of dawn to do it, even if they despair of not being able to sleep longer, caress their wives, make love, play with their kids, or just lie around listening to the radio, the bathroom always brighter and the smell of toast always more desirable on those mornings, guys who hope, then, to be part of this strange club, and who would have paid good money, even elbowed their way in to be chosen by Harfang – "pointed out" was the provisional term – because Harfang, suddenly aware of their presence, would point his index at them and tilt his head to the side to evaluate their physical constitution, making sure he had here a possible rival, and with a strange smile twisting his face, he would ask: so, you like biking?

Pedalling along at Harfang's side, following on his wheels for a few hours was worth facing their furious wives who found themselves alone with the kids on Sunday until the middle of the afternoon, their spitefully mocking remarks – don't worry dear, I know you're just making sacrifices for your family – was worth suffering their reproaches – you only think of yourself – and their vexing phrases when they looked them up and down, evaluating their paunches – careful you don't have a heart attack! worth coming home crimson, broken, legs barely holding up their bodies anymore and backsides so sore they dreamed of a sitz bath but sank into the first couch in their path, or into their beds, a well-deserved nap – and this arrogated rest, of course, set off the wrath of the wives again, who looped a lament about the selfishness of men, their foolhardy ambition, their submissiveness, their fear of growing old, raising their arms to the sky and exclaiming out loud, or planting their hands flat on their hips with elbows wide, stomachs out, and tormenting them, an Italian comedy – and once the men had recovered from their effort, it was worth it to linger at the computer for the urgent purchase of a chamois from a specialised site, matching shorts and all the right gear, ending up shouting shut up! at the woman grousing at the other end of the apartment, ending up making her cry; and it's a little surprising, really, that there wasn't a single woman who supported this masculine endeavour, not a single one who, whether careerist or simply compliant, encouraged her husband to mount a bike and follow Harfang along the paths in the Chevreuse Valley, to parade wingèd, light, hardy, yes, not a single one was fooled, and when they talked among themselves, deploring the insidious requisitioning of their husbands, they would sometimes cite Lysistrata, planning to go on strike for sex so that the men might stop their servile antics, or they might fall down laughing as they described their partners done in after the race, and in the end it was funny, fine, they should go if it makes them happy, they should wear themselves out, allies and adversaries, favourites and competitors, and soon not a single one of the women gets up at six in the morning to make coffee and hold it out to her husband with a loving hand, they all stay in bed, curled up in the duvet, dishevelled, warm and moaning.

The last time Marthe Carrare heard Harfang speak, he was giving a brilliant report on the success of Cyclosporine in anti-rejection treatments that had revolutionised transplants in the early 1980s, summing up the history of this immunosuppressive in twelve minutes – a product that lowers the immune defences in the recipient and reduces the risk of rejection of the transplanted organ – at the end of which he ran a hand through his hair and pushed back the famous white lock that excused him from having to repeat his family name, don't wear it out, and said, abruptly, any questions? counted one, two, three in his head, and concluded his talk by alluding to the end of heart transplantations, their coming obsolescence, because it was finally time to consider artificial hearts, marvels of technology invented and developed in a French laboratory – authorisation had been given to conduct the first tests in several countries, including Poland, Slovenia, Saudi Arabia, and Belgium. The bioprosthesis, weighing nine hundred grams, was developed over the course of twenty years by an internationally renowned French surgeon, and would be implanted in patients with severe heart failure in life-threatening situations. This conclusion disconcerted the room, a murmur rumbled through the audience, waking the dozers – the idea of the cardiac prosthesis that would purge the organ of its symbolic power, and even though most of the heads nodded toward spiral notebooks in order to record Harfang's words in telegraphic style, there were a few that shook side to side, unsettled and vaguely upset, and a few attentive individuals could be seen sliding a hand beneath their jacket, behind their tie, under their shirt, and holding it against their heart to feel it beating.

The kick-off has happened and the continuous murmur emanating from the stadium has grown to a roar that sounds at regular intervals – a shot on goal, a member of the opposition suddenly threatening, an elaborate play, a violent clash, a goal. Marthe Carrare leans back in her chair – the donor's organs have been distributed, the routes established, the teams formed, everything's on track. And Remige has it under control. As long as there's no unpleasant surprise during the harvesting, she thinks, as long as the physiognomy of the organs doesn't reveal anything that the scans, the ultrasounds and the analyses couldn't see or even suspect. She'd love to have one little smoke, with a beer and a good cheeseburger with barbeque sauce; she chews faster so she can squeeze out the last atom of nicotine from her gum, the memory of a taste, an odour, even faded, thinks of the security guard who must be following the game, leaning over a portable screen, his pack of Marlboro Lights within arm's reach.

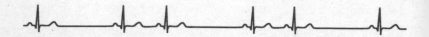

AS IT HAPPENS, CORDELIA OWL IS SHAKING A PACK OF CIGA-
rettes at this same moment while the doors of the lift slide closed,
signing to Revol through the progressively narrow opening, I'm going
down for a break, five minutes, then her own face appears in soft
focus against the metallic wall that isn't exactly a mirror but gives a
basic outline – the supple skin and shining eyes are gone, the sparkling trail of the sleepless night, that beauty, still aroused: her face has
turned as milk turns, features slumping, complexion clouded, an
olive-grey tugging at the khaki in the circles under her eyes, and the
marks on her neck have darkened. Once she's alone in the lift, she
sticks the cigarettes back into a pocket, takes her phone out of the
other, quick glance, still nothing, checks that the indicators are working, trembles, looks closer, oh, no network, not even the tiniest little
stream, the tiniest little glimmer, and hope finds her again, he must
have tried to call without being able to get through, and once she's on
the first floor, she runs toward a side exit door reserved for hospital
personnel, pushes the metal crossbar, and there she is outside, three
or four others smoking there, hopping from foot to foot in the compact cold, on the whitish square traced by the neon sign, orderlies and
a nurse she doesn't recognise, and the air is so freezing that it's impos-

sible to tell the tobacco smoke from the carbonic gas they exhale together. She turns her phone off and on again, that old story of starting over from scratch, of finding out for sure. Her bare arms go visibly blue, and soon all of her extremities are shaking. You guys have service here? She turns to the group, the voices are superimposed over each other, yeah, there is, I have service, me too, and once her device is restarted, she looks at it – she carries out these steps in disbelief, sure now that nothing has been left for her in her mailbox, sure that she has to stop thinking about it in order for something to happen.

Network in abundance, not a peep. She lights a cigarette. One of the guys in front of her tosses out you're in the I.C.U., right? He's a tall ginger, brush cut with an earring in his left ear and long hands with reddened fingers, short nails. Yeah, Cordelia answers, lowering her little trembling chin, she's sapped of strength, numb goosebumps, belly hurting from shivering beneath her thin shirt, she grips her cigarette tightly, smokes like someone who's lost, eyes suddenly burning, eyes crying, the guy looks at her, smiling, hey, you okay? what's going on? Nothing, she answers, nothing, I'm just cold, but the guy has come closer, the I.C.U.'s hard, eh, you see some crazy things, don't you? Cordelia sniffs and takes a drag, no, I'm fine, it's the cold, really, and I'm tired. Tears run down her cheeks, slow, tinted with mascara, tears of a little girl who's sobering up.

Everything bright and burning that had lashed about inside her, the full speed ahead lightness, playful and fierce, the queenly step that she still had this afternoon in the corridors of the I.C.U., all of this takes on water at a rapid rate and sways inside her brain, heavy, soaking: by dint of being twenty-three, she was twenty-eight, by dint of being twenty-eight, she was thirty-one; time cavorted while she cast a cold glance over her existence, a glance that brutally stripped each area of her life, one after the other – damp studio apartment where cockroaches proliferate and mould sprouts in the joints between tiles, bank loan that sucks up luxuries, hell-or-high-water friendships reconfigured, peripheralised, as newly created families spring up, polarised over cradles that leave her unmoved, days saturated with stress and girls' nights out spent on the sidelines but impeccably epilated, gossiping in dreary lounge bars, a bevy of available females and forced laughs which she always ends up joining, pusillanimous, opportunistic; or else the rare sexual episode on a cruddy mattress, against the oily soot of a parking lot door, guys who are often clumsy, rushed, cheap – in short, not very loving – copious amounts of alcohol to give a lustre to the whole thing; the only encounter that sets her heart to beating is a guy who lifts a lock of her hair to light her cigarette, brushes her temple and earlobe, and takes the art of appearing suddenly to a whole new level – and in fact he will appear at any moment, totally impossible to predict, as though he were always standing hidden behind a lamppost and would suddenly stick his head out to surprise her in the golden light of the end of the day, calling late at night from a café nearby, or walking toward her in the morning from the corner of the street, and always vanishing in the end, the great disappearing act, before coming back again the next time – it's the great scouring, nothing can resist, not even her face, not even her body that she takes care of all the same – women's magazines, tubes of slimming cream and that hour of floor bar in a freezing room at the Docks Vauban rec centre – she is single and disgraced, bitterly disappointed, she stamps her feet with her teeth chattering while disillusion ravages her land and her hinterland, darkens faces, rots gestures, skews intentions; it swells, proliferates, pollutes the rivers and the forests, contaminates the deserts, corrupts the groundwater, tears the petals from the flowers and sullies the fur of the animals, it stains the ice floes above the Arctic Circle and defiles the daybreak, smears the most beautiful poems with a viscous gloom, it pillages the planet and everything that populates it from the Big Bang to the rockets of the future, and stirs up the whole world, this world that rings hollow: this disenchanted world.

I'm gonna head in, she tosses her butt to the ground, crushes it with the toe of her canvas flat, the tall ginger watches her, you feeling better? She nods her head, I'm fine, see you later, does a half-turn, hurries inside the building, and the path back is an interlude that she uses to gather herself up again before getting back to the department, where work is intensifying at this hour: edginess of the evening, restless patients, last treatments before nighttime, last intravenous drips, last pills, and this harvesting that will happen in a few hours – Revol had come to ask her if she could replace someone at the last minute, extend her shift and stay on in the O.R., an exceptional request, she had said yes.

She takes a detour past the café to pick up a tomato soup from the automatic distributor, we see her walking through the icy lobby, skinny little thing with a tense jaw, and later hitting the machine with her fist to speed up the flow, the soup is foul and so boiling hot that the cup deforms in her hand, but she drinks it in one go, immediately warmed, when suddenly she sees them passing before her – the father and the mother, the parents of the patient from room seven, the young man whose catheter she had inserted earlier this afternoon, the one who is dead and whose organs will be harvested tonight, it's them; she follows with her eyes their slow walk toward the tall glass doors, leans against a pillar so she can see them better: the glass wall has become a mirror at this hour, they're reflected there the way ghosts are reflected in the surface of ponds on winter nights; they are a shadow of themselves, you might say to describe them, and the banality of this expression would be less a reference to their internal disintegration than an affirmation of what they still were only this morning – a man and a woman standing in the world; seeing them walk side by side over the ground varnished with cold light, it would be clear to everyone that from now on these two were following a new trajectory, begun just a few hours earlier – already they didn't entirely live in the same world as Cordelia and the other inhabitants of the earth, but were growing distant, withdrawing, moving toward another realm, which might have been the place where those who had lost a child could survive, for a short time, together and inconsolable.

Cordelia keeps their silhouettes in her frame of vision as they diminish at the edge of the parking lot, disappear into the night, then she lets out a cry, pushes off from the pillar, shakes herself like a colt, grabs her phone, her face falls back into place and colours return, and in an incredible pendulum movement, she enacts an interior about-face that revives her, finds a momentum that signifies recovery, speedily dials the number of the man who disappeared at five in the morning, surprising herself with this action, plinking dexterously on the keys, as though she wanted both to rid herself of the thing and to confront the subjugation she's been confined to by her sadness, as though she wanted to counter the morbidity that assails her and remember the possibility of love. One, two, three rings, and then it's the guy's voice saying in three languages leave me a message – I love you, and she hangs up, curiously reinvigorated, relieved of a weight: she suddenly has her whole life ahead of her once again, tells herself she always cries when she's tired, and that she must be low in magnesium.

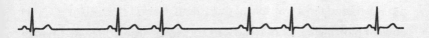

LOU. THEY HADN'T CALLED LOU, HADN'T TRIED TO TALK TO HER, hadn't thought of her, except to ask that her name be said into her brother's ear at the moment when they stopped his heart. But Lou, this little seven-year-old girl, her distress at seeing her mother leave for an emergency at the hospital, her waiting, her aloneness – all this, they hadn't thought about it, and although it's true they were confronted with the cyclonic charge of death, drafted into tragedy, they don't try to make any excuses, and they fly into a panic when they see the neighbour's number on Marianne's mobile, along with the notification of a voicemail they don't have the strength to listen to, and now Marianne presses on the accelerator, murmuring toward the windshield, we're coming, we're coming home.

The bells ring at the top of the Church of Saint-Vincent and the sky has the rumpled look of a melting candle. It's six-thirty when they climb the turns of the Ingouville coast, plunge into the building's underground parking lot, the return; we'll stay together tonight, Marianne said as she turned off the engine – but could they possibly have had the strength to separate that night, Marianne staying here with Lou, Sean going back to his two-room apartment rented in a rush last November, in Dollemard? Marianne struggles to get the key into the lock, can't manage to engage the mechanism, the metallic jiggling goes on inside the hole while Sean paces behind her, and when the door finally opens they're off balance and topple inside. Don't turn on any lights, just collapse side by side on to the couch that they found on the side of a country road one rainy day, wrapped up like a candy in a transparent tarp, and around them the walls veer toward blotting paper now, absorb this scrap-iron coffee that signals the end of the day: in the few paintings hanging there, other figures appear, other forms, the furniture swells, the patterns on the carpet are erased, the room is like a shiny piece of paper left too long in the basin of liquid developer, and this transmutation – this progressive silting-up, the darkening of all that surrounds them – hypnotises them; the world around them absconds; the physical suffering they feel isn't enough to lash them to the real, this is a nightmare, we have to wake up from it sometime, this is what Marianne says to herself as she stares at the ceiling – and if in fact Simon came home, here, now, if he in his turn made the lock click and then came into the apartment, slamming the door behind him with this abrupt loud gesture that was typical of his entrances, inevitably setting off his mother's shout, Simon stop slamming that door! if he turned up in this moment, surfboard under his arm squeaking inside its cover, hair damp, face and hands bluish from the cold, exhausted by the sea, Marianne would be the first to believe it, would get up, go toward him, offer him eggs with paprika, pasta, something hot and invigorating, yes, she wouldn't see a ghost, she would just see the return of her child.

*

Marianne's hand reaches out to touch Sean's, or his arm, or his thigh, any place on his body it can reach, but this hand stretches out into emptiness, because Sean just got up, shrugged off his parka, I'm going down to get Lou. He starts walking toward the door but now the doorbell rings, he opens it, Marianne lets out a cry, she's here.

She's excited, comes running into the apartment, has pulled a long multicoloured T-shirt on over her clothes, tied a scarf into her hair and someone has attached two iridescent tulle butterfly wings to her back with the help of some Velcro – she too has straight black hair, olive skin, and deep eyes, delicately drawn – suddenly she pulls up short in front of her father, surprised to see him in a sweater inside the apartment, are you back? Behind her, the neighbour stays on the doorstep but leans a head inside the apartment – a giraffe's manoeu-vre – her face is an open sky of a question: Sean, have you come back? We just got here – he stops his sentence short, doesn't want to talk. In front of him, Lou hops from foot to foot as she rummages in her bag, finally hands him a piece of white paper, I did a drawing for Simon, she moves forward into the living room, and finding her mother cap-sized on the couch, asks abruptly: where's Simon? is he still at the hospital? Without waiting for a reply, she turns around, rushes down the hall, wings vibratile and step pounding, we hear her open a door, call out to her brother, then other doors slam, and this same name is called again, and then the child reappears in the doorway, in front of her two parents standing there, distraught, waiting, unable to speak, unable to say anything other than Lou, softly, while the neighbour, pale, backs up into the stairwell, making a sign with her index finger, showing she's understood, doesn't want to bother them, closes the door behind her.

The child is facing her parents while the day declines in the west, slowly plunging the city into darkness, and now they are only silhou-

159

ettes. Marianne and Sean come closer, the little girl doesn't shy away, remains silent, eyes devouring the darkness – pupils pinpoints white as kaolin clay – Sean picks her up, then Marianne wraps her arms around them both – the three bodies commingled eyelids closed like on port monuments in the south of Ireland in memory of the people drowned – then they sit back down on the couch, moving diagonally without coming unstuck, a Roman triad that protects itself from the outside, here they curl up inside their breath and the scent of their skin – the little girl smells like brioche and Haribo – and it's the first time they catch their breath since the terrible news, the first time they nest inside a cavity of withdrawal at the heart of their devastation, and if you come a little closer, if you are soft and silent, you can hear their hearts together, pumping the life that's left, and banging, tumultuous, as though sensors have been placed on the valves or against the arteries and are emitting infrasonic lines, those lines that stretch out into space, rushing through material, sure, precise, reaching Japan, the Seto Sea, an island, a wild beach and that wood cabin where they archive the beatings of human hearts, those cardiac imprints collected the world over, deposited or recorded here by the rare few who have made the long journey, and while Marianne's and Sean's hearts beat in rhythm, the little girl's hammers, until she suddenly sits up, the skin of her forehead covered with a film of sweat: why are we sitting in the dark? A cat, she slides out of her parents' embrace, walks around the room turning all the lamps on one by one and then turns back toward them and declares: I'm hungry.

Alert sounds multiply, signalling the messages flowing into voice-mail boxes – they have to think about talking now, about telling people, this is another ordeal to face. Marianne goes out on to the balcony – she still has her coat on – lights a cigarette, prepares herself to call for news of Chris and Johan, finds a message from Juliette, suddenly doesn't know what to do anymore, scared to speak and scared to hear, scared that it will get stuck in her throat, because with Juliette it meant a lot – Simon had introduced her begrudgingly last December, on a Wednesday, they were in the kitchen when Marianne had come home at an unusual time, he hadn't said "this is my mother," just "Juliette, Marianne," immediately murmuring let's go, we have things to do, while Marianne was starting to engage her in conversation, so you're in the same school as Simon? staggered to discover that this was what she looked like, the girl who had taken up residency in her son's heart, and she was an original enough model that Marianne would be surprised, didn't look like anyone, least of all a groupie from the beach – she was frail, flat-chested, with a strange sweet little face, eyes that took up almost the whole thing, ears with multiple piercings, gap teeth and that pale blonde hair cut like Jean Seberg in *Breathless*; that first day she was wearing pale-pink skinny cords over bright green high-tops, a Jacquard twinset under a red raincoat; Simon had waited with irritation while she answered Marianne, then had led her toward the door, pulling her by the elbow, and later he had started to leave her name lying around here and there, scattering it in the middle of the rare stories he consented to tell, until hers ended up rivalling the names of his friends and those of surf spots on the Pacific; he's changing, Marianne had thought, because Simon had started abandoning McDonalds for that Irish pub that smelled like wet dog, was reading Japanese novels, went to collect driftwood on the beach, and sometimes did homework with her, chemistry, physics, biology, subjects he excelled in, not her, and one evening Marianne heard him describe the form of the wave to her: look (he must have been drawing a diagram), the swell moves toward the shore, it tautens as the water shallows, they call that the shoaling zone, that's where the waves crest, sometimes it's really violent, then the swell reaches the breaker zone, that can cover up to a hundred metres if the bottom of the spot is rocky, those are the point breaks, and then the waves break in the surf zone but continue to move toward the shore, get it? (she must have said yes, nodding her little chin), and at the end of the ride, if you're really lucky, there's a girl there on the beach, a cute girl in a red raincoat; they talked late into the night while the rest of the house slept, and maybe they even whispered I love you to each other then, not knowing what they were saying but only that they were saying it to each other, that was the important thing – because Juliette, she was Simon's heart.

Marianne holds herself up on the balcony, fingers sealed by the cold to the metal railing. From this promontory, she overlooks the city, the estuary, the sea. Streetlights with curved covers lit by orange bulbs highlight the main streets, the port and the coastline, cold flames creating powdery Payne's grey haloes in the sky, traffic lights signalling the entrance to the port at the end of the long jetty, while beyond the edge of coastline it's black tonight, not a single stranded boat, not a blink, just a slow, pulsing mass – the shadows. What will Juliette's love become once Simon's heart starts beating in another, unknown body? what will become of all that filled this heart, its affects slowly deposited in strata from the first day, or injected here and there in a rush of enthusiasm or a fit of anger, his friendships and his aversions, his resentments, his vehemence, his grave and tender inclinations? What will become of the electric surges that coursed so strongly through his heart as the wave came near? What will become of this overflowing heart, full, too full, what will become of it? Marianne looks at the yard, the still pines, the windows of the apartments across the way that pour their warm light out into the darkness, the blushings of living rooms and the yellows of kitchens – topaz, saffron, mimosa, and this Naples yellow, even more dazzling behind the steam of the windowpanes – and the rectangle of green of a stadium field, fluorescent, soon it will be time for Sunday dinner, that other kind of meal, self-serve and folding trays, bread pudding, crepes, hard-boiled eggs, a ritual signifying that just for tonight she wouldn't cook anything, and then there they were, sprawled out before a football game, or a movie they could watch together, and Simon's profile was cut out clearly in the light of the lamp. She turns around, Sean is there, watching her, forehead pressed to the bay window, and Lou, lying on the couch, has fallen asleep.

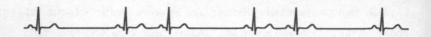

ANOTHER CALL, ANOTHER TELEPHONE THAT TREMBLES ON A table and a hand that picks it up – this one has a ring of gold, a large, dull ring, veined with spirals – another voice that follows the vibrational rumble – this one has been through the meat grinder, it's plain to see, "Harfang surg." came up on the mobile screen – hello? And another piece of news – it's visible on the face of the woman who's listening, emotion races beneath the epidermis, and then the features contract once again, furl.

– We have a heart. A compatible heart. A team is leaving immediately to harvest it. Come now. The transplant will happen tonight. You'll be taken into O.R. around midnight.

She hangs up, she's out of breath. Turns toward the only window in the room and gets up to open it, pressing down on the desk with both hands in order to lift herself up, the three steps that follow are difficult, and the effort to turn the handle is even more so. Winter gathers in the window frame – a hardened panel, translucent and glacial. It vitrifies the noises of the street that ring out, isolated, like the murmur of evening in a provincial village, neutralises the cry of the skytrain that brakes at the entrance to Chevaleret station, garrottes odours and lays a film of ice over her face, she shivers, slowly brings her eyes to the other side of Vincent-Auriol boulevard, straight across, touching the windows of the building that houses the cardiology department of the Pitié-Salpêtrière hospital, where she'd been for tests three days before – the state of her heart had greatly deteriorated, this is why the cardiologist had called the Agency of Biomedicine to place her in a priority position on the list of recipients. She thinks about what she's experiencing, now, in this second; she says to herself: I'm saved, I'm going to live; she says to herself: someone somewhere died a violent death; she says to herself: it's now, it's tonight; she feels the gravity of the news; she wishes this flash of the present would never pull back to become a representation, that it would stay as an afterglow; she says to herself: I am mortal.

She breathes in the winter for a long moment, eyes closed: the bluish planet drifts in a fold of the cosmos, suspended silently in a gaseous material, the forest is starred with rectilinear rays, red ants stir at the foot of the trees in a sticky jelly, the garden dilates – mosses and stones, grass after rain, heavy branches, scratch of the palm tree – the cambered city encloses the multitude, children in bunk beds open their eyes in the darkness; she imagines her heart, morsel of dark red flesh, seeping, fibrous, all its various pipes, this organ beset by necrosis, this organ that's failing. She closes the window again. She has to get ready.

Nearly a year that Claire Méjan has lived in this two-room apartment rented sight unseen, the words "Pitié-Salpêtrière" and "second floor" having been enough to make her sign a cheque immediately for an exorbitant amount to the guy at the agency – it's dirty, small, and dark, the cornice of the balcony on the third floor shading her window like a hat brim. But she doesn't have a choice. That's what it is to be sick, she tells herself, to not have a choice – her heart doesn't give her the choice anymore.

It's myocarditis. She found out three years ago during an appointment in the cardiology department at Pitié-Salpêtrière. Eight days before, the flu again, and she poked at the crackling fireplace with a blanket over her shoulders while in the garden snapdragons and foxgloves bent under the wind. She had been to see a doctor at the Fontainebleu, complaining of fever, of aches and fatigue, but had neglected to tell him about these occasional palpitations, this pain in her chest, this shortness of breath that came with every effort, getting these signs confused with lassitude, winter, a lack of light, a kind of general exhaustion. She left the appointment armed with anti-flu meds; she would stay in her room and work from her bed. A few days later, after dragging herself to Paris to see her mother, she goes into a state of shock: her blood pressure drops, her skin goes pale, cold, and sweaty. She's taken to emergency sirens wailing – cliché of an American T.V. series – they revive her, and then the first tests begin. Straightaway a blood test confirms inflammation, and then they examine her heart. A flurry of tests follows: the electrocardiogram detects a rhythm anomaly, the X-ray shows a slightly dilated heart, the echocardiography finally confirms heart failure. Claire stays in hospital, she's transferred to cardiology, where the tests become more and more specialised. The coronary angiography is normal, which rules out the possibility of a heart attack, so they proceed to biopsy her heart: Claire is pricked inside the cardiac muscle via the jugular. A few hours later, the results of the biopsy let drop a hostile hendeca-syllable: inflammation of the myocardium.

The treatment covers two fronts: heart failure – the heart is

166

exhausted, it's not beating efficiently anymore – and irregularities in the rhythm. Mandatory rest is prescribed for Claire, zero physical effort, plus antiarrhythmic agents and beta blockers, and a defibrillator is implanted in order to prevent sudden death. They treat the viral infection at the same time, prescribing powerful immuno-suppressants and anti-inflammatories. But the illness persists, grows more serious – it invades the muscle tissue, the heart grows more and more distended, and each second carries a lethal risk. The organ's deterioration is judged to be irreversible: they have to operate. A transplant. Another human heart implanted in place of her own – the hand gestures of the doctor, there again, mime the surgical act. In the end, it's the only option.

She goes home that same night – her youngest son has come to pick her up at the hospital, he drives on the way back. You're going to say yes, right? he murmurs softly. She nods mechanically – she's crushed. When they reach her house at the edge of the forest, this fairy-tale house where she lives alone now, her children grown and gone, she goes upstairs to her room and lies down on her back, stares at the ceiling: fear pins her to the bed, irradiating future days and leaving no room for possible loopholes – fear of death and fear of pain, fear of the operation, of the post-operation treatments, fear her body will reject it and that everything will begin all over again, fear of the intrusion of a stranger's body inside her own, and fear of becoming a Chimera – of not being herself anymore.

She'll have to move – she's taking a risk, living in this village sixty-five kilometres from Paris, far from the major highways.

Claire hates the new apartment right from the start. Overheated in summer as in winter, lights on in the middle of the day, the noise. Last airlock before the operating room, she envisions it more as the ante-chamber of death, believing she'll die there without having been able to leave because even though she's not bedridden, she is trapped, every exfiltration requiring a superhuman effort, each step on the staircase increasing her pain, each movement causing the sensation that her heart is separating from the rest of her body, unhooking from inside her ribcage, tumbling down in pieces, a dislocation that makes her into this shaky, claudicant creature, on the edge of break-ing. Day after day space contracts around her, places a quota on her gestures, restricts her movements, a shrinking of everything as though her head were stuck in a plastic bag, a nylon, something fibrous that suffocates her and coats her life in a sticky murk. A shadow comes over her. One night when her youngest son comes to see her she tells him that waiting to contain the heart of a dead person disturbs her, it's a strange state of affairs, you know, and it's wearing me out.

At the beginning, she's reluctant to really settle in – whether she lives or dies she won't stay here, it's just temporary – but still she puts on a brave face. The first weeks in this apartment change her relationship to time. It's not that time has changed speed, slowed down by paraly-sis, the anguish of suspension, or all that she's prevented from doing, nor is it that it stagnates like blood stagnates in Claire's lungs – no, it just crumbles away in a dismal continuity. The alternation of day and night soon has no caesura – the constant dimness of rooms contrib-utes to this – and all she does is sleep, on the pretext of canalising the shock of this forced move. Little by little, her two older sons instate Sunday as visiting day, which makes her sad without knowing exactly why. They sometimes reproach her for her lack of enthusiasm – right across from the Pitié, after all, it doesn't get better than that, they say, without a trace of irony. The youngest one, though, still turns up at any time, and takes her in his arms for long moments – he's a head taller than her.

Dreary winter, cruel spring – she doesn't see the greening of the forest, the colours that explode again, strong, and she misses the undergrowth, the golden stumps and the ferns, the light that plumbs space in vertical rays, the multitude of sounds, the foxglove scattered in the partial shade on secret paths behind the mountains. Desperate summer. She grows weak – you need a routine, say those who stop in to see her, meals at fixed times, a daily framework, they hammer out the refrain; they find her depressed, elsewhere, uncertain and a little alarming, her dark-eyed blonde beauty altering, corroded by anxiety and the lack of the outdoors – her hair is dull, her eyes are glassy, she has bad breath and lives in loose clothes. Her two eldest try to find someone to take care of her, a homecare worker who'll come to do housework, shopping, and could monitor treatments. When she catches wind of this scheme, she bristles, enraged, are they trying to spear the little bit of freedom she has left? House arrest, she stammers, white and bitter, can't stand it anymore, the view the healthy have of sickness.

A first call comes to her on the night of the fifteenth of August, the window's open, it's eight in the evening, they're suffocating in the room – it's the Pitié, we have a heart, it's tonight, it's now, always the same antiphony; she's not ready, puts her fork down on her untouched plate, looks at her family pressed in around her, together for her birthday, her fiftieth, they've folded their elbows along their sides like birds' wings, her mother, her three boys, the young woman who lives with the oldest and their little boy, all sitting frozen except for the child with garnet eyes, I'm going, I have to go, chairs topple, champagne flutes vibrate, things splash and spill, a suitcase with toothpaste and face mist is buckled closed, they go down the stairs with that hurried slowness that causes them to stumble and snap at each other – the sorbets in the kitchen are forgotten, the health card is forgotten, the telephone is forgotten – then it's sticky pavement, smoky sky, people hanging from windows, a bare-chested guy walking his dog, a little boy running on the pavement, caught by his mother, tourists that consult their map at the exit from the Metro, and finally the hospital fringed with little lights, the front desk, the scrubbed room where she waits again, sitting on the edge of this bed that she won't ever get into, because in the end there's a scuffling in the corridor, footsteps hammer the ground, and Harfang appears, suddenly there before her, pale and blunt, red-rimmed eyes: we've had to refuse the heart.

She listens to him explaining his decision, lets nothing show – the heart is no good, small and poorly perfused, it's a useless risk, we'll have to wait longer. Harfang believes she's in shock, disappointed, crushed by false hope, but really she's just stunned, dazed, with only one thought in mind – to get out of here; her feet hang in the void, her buttocks slide imperceptibly toward the edge of the bed, she lands gently on the ground, then pulls herself up straight, I'm going home. Outside, her sons kick in the bushes that release their burning dust, her mother bursts into tears in the arms of the youngest son, the eldest's partner continues to chase the little boy who doesn't want to go to sleep, and everything breaks down. The group leaves, back the way they came, no appetite now, impossible to sit down again to the meal they'd left; but they could drink, a rosé champagne in bubbly flutes and Claire who holds her full glass out over the table smiling, beautiful now, don't take it to heart! You're not funny, you know, her youngest son murmurs.

And then time changes character again, it regains its shape. Or rather it takes the exact shape of waiting: it hollows and stretches out. From now on the hours have only one use – to be available, for the event of the transplant to be able to take place, a heart could appear at any moment, I have to be alive, I have to be ready. Minutes become malleable, seconds ductile and then autumn arrives, and Claire resolves to have her books and her lamps brought to these thirty square metres, her youngest son sets up Wi-Fi for her, she buys a pull-out couch, a wooden table, gathers a few objects: she wants to start translating again.

In London, her editor greets this return gladly, sends her Charlotte Bronte's first collection, poems published with her sisters under masculine pen-names: Currer, Ellis, and Acton Bell. Autumn passes in a freezing cottage battered by winds where three sisters and a brother write and read together by the light of a few candles, united by books, restless, exalted, tortured geniuses who invent worlds, beat through the heath, drink litres of tea, and smoke opium. Their intensity is infectious and Claire perks up. Each day of translating delivers its lot of attempts, sets down a few pages; the weeks pass and a working rhythm is established, as though it were a matter of synchronising the wait – which becomes clearer as the state of her heart degrades – with another timeline, that of poems to translate. She sometimes has the feeling she's substituting a fluid back-and-forth movement for the painful contractions of her ailing organ, the come and go that happens between her native French and her second language, English, and that this rotary movement carves a crevice in her in the form of a cradle, a new cavity – she had to learn another language to truly come to know her own, and now she asks herself whether this other heart will allow her to know herself even more deeply: I'll make room for you, my heart, I'll clear a space for you.

On Christmas Eve a man resurfaces with an armful of purple foxgloves, digitalis, that he places on her bed. She's known him since she was a child, they grew up together – lovers, friends, brother and sister, accomplices, they are nearly everything a man and a woman can be to one another.

Claire smiles, surprises are risky, I have a heart condition, you know. Indeed, she has to sit down and recover while he takes off his coat. The flowers are from her home, she can smell it. They're toxic, did you know that? she says, pointing at them. The kind you forbid children to touch, breathe in, gather, taste – she remembers contemplating her fingers powdered with fuchsia, fascinated, alone on the path, and the word "poison" that swelled above her little girl head when she brought them toward her mouth. The man slowly plucks a petal and places it in the hollow of her hand: here, look. The colour of the petal is so vivid that you would think it was fake, made of plastic; it trembles in her palm and grows covered with microscopic creases as he tells her: the digitalis contained in the flowers slows and regularises the movements of the heart, it supports cardiac contraction, it's a good molecule for you.

That night, she falls asleep with the flowers. The man undresses her with care, unfolds the petals one by one and places them on her naked skin like the scales of a fish, a vegetal puzzle forming a ceremonial cloak: he takes care to perfect it, murmuring from time to time, don't move, can you do that for me, and meanwhile she sinks into a cataleptic state of delight, ornamented and tended to like a queen. When she wakes, it's still dark, but the children are already tumbling around in the apartment upstairs, letting out shouts, their heels hammering the floor, they're running to tear open the paper of presents that had appeared in the night near the ectoplasmic Christmas tree. Her friend is gone. She shakes the petals off her body and uses them to make a salad that she dresses with truffle oil and balsamic.

A T-shirt, a few pairs of underwear, two nightshirts, a pair of slippers, toiletries, her laptop, her phone, the various chargers. Her medical file – the administrative forms, the last tests, and these big stiff envelopes containing X-rays, scans, and MRIs. She's glad to be alone while she packs her bag, to go down the stairs with a careful step, to take her time outside. She crosses the boulevard on a diagonal, trying to catch the eyes of the drivers who brake before her, listens to the burning rails vibrating above her head, she wishes she might meet an animal – ideally a tiger, or a barn owl, its facial disc in the shape of a heart, but a stray dog would do just fine, or some simply marvellous bees. She is more terrified than she's ever been, she's anaesthetised by terror. I should probably call, she says to herself as she enters the hospital grounds, she scrolls through to her sons' numbers, sends them a text – it's happening, tonight – calls her mother who's probably already asleep, and last, her friend of the foxgloves on the other side of the world, signals that are emanations of this present moment and that stretch out long in the fabric of time, she turns around once more, looks hard at the window of her apartment, and suddenly all the hours she's spent waiting behind that wall of glass condense into a sliver of time and converge in the back of her skull at the very instant she passes through the hospital gates, quick snap of the fingers that sends her into the inner walls, along the paved ribbon that runs past the buildings, then it's a left turn, she enters the cardiology institute, a lobby, two lifts – she holds herself back from thinking she must choose the one that will bring her luck – fourth floor and this corridor lit like a space station, the nurses' desks walled in glass, and Harfang standing there, white coat clean and buttoned, white lock smoothed back from his forehead: I've been waiting for you.

174

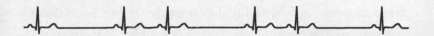

THE MARGHERITA SPLATS AGAINST THE APARTMENT WALL AND falls to the carpet, leaving the trace of a Neapolitan sunset above the television. The young woman appraises her throw with a satisfied eye and turns back to the pile of white boxes on the counter of the open kitchen, lifts the lid of a second perfectly quadrangular box, slides the burning disc of the Supreme on to her palm, turns to face the wall, elbow bent, hand held as a tray, and with a quick extension of her arm, projects it between the room's two windows, a new action painting, slices of pepperoni drawing a curious constellation on the wall. As she's preparing to break open the third box – a blistering Four-Cheese, she banks on the yellowish melted mix being a reliable adhesive paste – a man steps out of the bathroom, glistening, and then – sensing a threat – stops short in the doorway; seeing the young woman wind up for a gesture of propulsion in his direction, he drops to the floor, pure reflex, then rolls from his belly on to his back to observe her from a low angle. She smiles, turns away, eyes scanning her canvas, and then, taking care to target a new spot, she throws the pizza against the front door. Finally she steps over the stunned young man and goes to wash her hands behind the counter. The guy gets up, checks to make sure there are no spots on his clothes, and then takes

175

stock of the damages, turning slowly, a circular scope that brings him back to the woman stationed in front of the sink.

She's drinking a glass of water. Her pearly-white shoulders emerge from an undershirt with the green, white and red of the Squadra Azzurra, the low-cut neckline hinting at small breasts, free and light, her incredibly long legs extend from a pair of loose blue satiny shorts, and a fine film of sweat pearls above her mouth: she's beautiful as day, maxillaries pulsing beneath the skin of her jaw – fury – and doesn't even look at him as she crosses and uncrosses her long arms of an ancient beauty, low to high, in order to take off her tank top, useless now, revealing a splendid bust composed of various circles – breasts, areolae, nipples, belly, navel, top of the two globes of her buttocks – formed of various triangles pointing toward the ground – isosceles of the sternum, convex of the pubis, and concave of the lower back – crossed by various lines – the dorsal median that emphasises the division of the body into two identical halves, furrow reminiscent of the veining of the leaf and the butterfly's axis of symmetry – all punctuated by a small diamond at the crest of the sternum – the dark hollow at the base of the throat – altogether a collection of perfect forms whose balanced proportion and ideal arrangement he admires, his professional eye valuing the anatomical exploration of the human body above all else, and of this one in particular, delighting in its auscultation, detecting with passion the least disharmony in the elaboration, the smallest flaw, the tiniest discrepancy, the twist of scoliosis above the lumbar vertebrae, this spore of a beauty mark under the armpit, these calluses between the toes at the place where the foot is compressed inside the point of the high-heeled shoe, and the light strabismus of the eyes, coquetterie in one eye when she's lacking sleep, and which gives her this distracted look, this air of a girl on the loose that he likes so much.

She pulls on a turtleneck, takes off her shorts to slide into a pair of skinny jeans, show's over, it seems, then puts on high-heeled boots and heads for the door that drips with grease, opens and slams it behind her without a single look back at the young man standing in the middle of the sullied apartment, who watches her go, relieved.

You'll be going to Le Havre hospital to harvest. It's a heart, and it's now. When he heard this phrase from Harfang's mouth, uttered just as he'd been imagining for months, short and curt, Virgilio Breva nearly lost his voice, the combination of joy and disappointment forming a bitter lump in his throat. Sure, he was on call, and although he was excited by his mission, the news couldn't come at a worse time – rare conjunction of two events that were impossible to miss: a France–Italy match and a desirous Rose at home. And he wondered for a long time why Harfang had bothered to call him in person, suspecting a kind of twisted desire to mock him on a historic evening, because Harfang knew he was a soccer fan – Virgilio had long used Sunday morning practices as a legitimate excuse to save himself from the bike excursions – torture, he would murmur, dumbfounded, seeing the swarm of polliwogs set off with their pointy helmets and multicoloured bike shorts, with Harfang at the centre, playing the queen.

Virgilio's in the back of the taxi heading for the Pitié-Salpêtrière, he pulls his fur-lined hood down to his shoulders and gets a hold of himself. He's all stirred up from the tension of the past hour when what he needs is to be in top form, be on top of his game as never before. Because tonight will be a big night, tonight will be *his* night.

The quality of the transplant depends upon the quality of the retrieval, that's the governing principle, and tonight he's on the front line.

It's time to pull yourself together, he thinks, interlacing his fingers in their leather gloves, it's time to call it off with this woman, this crazy broad, and to put self-preservation first, even if he has to deprive himself of her in order to do so, of her hyperactive body and the sparkle of her presence. He goes over the past hour with alarm, Rose surprising him at home when he had planned to go out and watch the game with others, then demanding, sweet but vaguely threatening, that they stay home to watch it together and order pizza, already equipped with a playful point in her favour – this azzurra soccer fan suit; the erotic tension between them coiling gradually with that other tension, war-like and upper case, of the match to come, a madly alluring mix that seeped potential happiness, and Harfang's call at the stroke of eight had pushed things to a fever pitch, the agitation going off the scale, penetrating the roof. He'd leapt to his feet immediately and answered I'm here, I'm ready, I'm on my way, avoiding Rose's eyes but exaggerating a tragic look – eyebrows in circumflex accents and bottom lip pulled up over the top one, oval of the chin lengthened sadly – a look meant to convey disaster, bad luck, bad dice, a look meant for Rose, grimacing for her at this moment, hand fanning the air, Guignolesque, a tragedian at the bazaar, while his eyes were radiating exultation – a heart! – she wasn't fooled. He backed off to take a shower, get dressed again in something clean and warm, and when he came out of the bathroom, things were already spiralling out of control. A magnificent and exhausting show, one that, now that he revisits it in slow motion, now that he perceives the logical majesty of it, does nothing but increase Rose's precellence, her incomparable splendour and her fiery temperament, the young woman releasing her fury in sovereign style and maintaining a royal mutism where so many others would have simply wailed. Splat! Splat! Splat! and the more he thinks about it, the more it becomes clear that breaking up with her would be folly, this beauty who is both highly inflammatory and entirely unique – he would never give her up, no matter what anyone said, those who took her for a madwoman, those who took her for "cray-cray" as they say, with a knowing glance, when really they would have given anything to touch that trapeze of warm skin at the back of her beautiful knee.

She had pushed open the door of the required class at the Pitié-Salpêtrière, beginning of the university year, the series of lectures during clerkship in the form of directed studies in a particular subject: the study of clinical cases. During long sessions, real case studies from the hospital or imagined, question-based scenarios were "re-enacted" for the students so they could practise their bedside manner, learn the movements of auscultation, train themselves to make a diagnosis, identify a pathology, and determine a treatment protocol. These practical sessions, structured around the patient–caregiver duo, took place in front of other students and sometimes required the presence of a larger group, in order to facilitate dialogue between different disciplines – the aim was to counteract a compartmentalization of medical specialties that cut up the human body into a collection of hermetically sealed knowledge and practices, leaving practitioners incapable of seeing the patient as a whole. But this new pedagogy – founded on simulation – aroused suspicion: the use of fiction in the process of acquiring scientific knowledge, the very idea of a re-enactment in the form of a game – they'd say, you be the doctor, and you be the patient – was enough to make the faculty directors sceptical. And yet they consented, acknowledging that this model combined material of a great richness, including subjectivity and emotion, and gave students a chance to work on that fragile exchange, the patient–doctor dialogue (even if it was falsified and displaced), that they needed to hear and learn to decode. In this role play, it was decided that the students would take on the role of the doctors in order to exercise their future function, and so actors were hired to play the patients.

They showed up after the appearance of a small ad in a weekly magazine for theatre professionals. Most of them were out-of-work actors, beginners full of promise or eternal second fiddles in T.V. shows, surveyors of commercial spots, doubles, extras, silhouettes, running from casting to casting just to make enough to pay the rent – usually a roommate situation in a neighbourhood in the northeast of Paris, or in a nearby suburb – or changing gears to become coaches for training sessions in sales techniques – door-to-door or elsewhere – and sometimes they even ended up taking part in guinea pig panels where they rented out their bodies, tasters of yogurt, testers of moisturising cream or anti-lice shampoo, experimenters of diuretic pills.

They were a multitude, they had to be selected. Medical professors who were also practitioners formed a jury – some of them theatre lovers – and they took no pains to hide it. When Rose entered the audition room and walked past the benches wearing platform sneakers, burgundy Adidas leggings, and a metallic sweater in sunset colours, there was a stir – didn't they recognise that body and that face from somewhere? They gave her a list of gestures and words in order to become a patient who'd rushed to the gynaecologist after discovering a suspicious lump in her left breast and, during the fifteen minutes that followed, her commitment to the role forced their admiration: she even stretched out topless on the floor of the room – tiles here, too – guiding the student's hand, there, there, it hurts,

180

yeah there; as the scene dragged on some discord ensued (and it's true that the student did exaggerate the length of his palpation, going back and forth from one breast to the other, always starting over, indifferent to the words of the dialogue, deaf to the essential information she was still giving him – among other things, that the pain got worse at the end of her menstrual cycle), until she finally sat up, face flushed, and slapped him soundly. Bravo, mademoiselle! She was congratulated, and hired on the spot.

From the very first days, Rose secretly flaunted the terms of the contract, considering that this job she'd landed as a "patient" for the duration of the university year would be a kind of training for herself, a chance to up her game, to increase the power of her art. She disdained commonplace pathologies (those she believed to be such), and instead hogged all the madness, hysteria, and melancholia, registers she excelled at – romantic heroine or enigmatic pervert – sometimes taking unexpected bifurcations from the original scenario with a nerve that stunned the psychiatrists and neurologists directing the sessions, and created some confusion among the students (they finally asked her to tone it down just a little); she tried her hand at drowning victims, suicidal patients, bulimics, erotomaniacs, and diabetics, liked doing a limp, a deformation (a case of Breton coxalgia gave rise to an interesting dialogue about consanguinity in the North Finistère – hunchbacks – she was able to mimic the rotation of vertebrae in the ribcage) and anything that required her to distort her body; she had fun playing a pregnant woman with premature contractions, but was less brilliant as a young mother describing the symptoms of a three-month-old infant – stress pearled on the forehead of the paediatric apprentice; superstitious, she turned down cancers.

And yet, she was never better than that day in December when she had to simulate angina. The renowned cardiologist who directed the session had described the pain to her in these terms: a bear is sitting on your thorax. Rose had widened her almond eyes in awe, a bear? She had to round up childhood emotions, the huge evil-smelling cage with grossly hewn plastic rocks, and the enormous animal, some five to seven hundred kilos, the triangular muzzle and close-set eyes, making it seem short-sighted, rusty fur dusted with sand, and the shouts of the children when it stood up on its back paws, two metres tall at its full height; she thought again of Ceaușescu's hunting scenes in the Carpathian Mountains – the bears rounded up by country folk, lured with buckets of food, emerging from the forest at the edge of the clearing where a wooden cabin was mounted on stilts, moving forward right into the frame of the window behind which a Securitate agent was loading the gun and offering it to the dictator (once the bear was close enough that he couldn't miss) – and, finally, she remembered a scene from *Grizzly Man*. Rose gathered momentum from the back of the room, walked toward the student who was her partner and then stopped – did she glimpse the animal, then, at the edge of some undergrowth, passing its head between two stalks of bamboo or swaying its hips on all fours, nonchalant, liquorice coat, lazily scratching a stump with its non-retractable claws before turning in her direction and standing up straight like a human? Did she see the cave-dwelling monster emerging from months of hibernation, stretching, warming up the fluids that had stopped inside its body, reactivating the drop of blood in its heart? Did she glimpse it rummaging through supermarket waste bins at twilight, growling with joy beneath an enormous moon? Or was she thinking of a different weight entirely – a man? Abruptly, she fell over backwards – the sound of her body falling caused a stir in the room – and in a convulsive tension, let out a shriek of pain that quickly became a silent gasp, and then she stopped breathing. Her rib cage seemed to flatten and hollow like a basin as her face swelled, slowly turning red, lips pressed tight together and going white, eyes rolling back in her head, while her limbs began to fibrillate as though shot through with an electric current. Such realism was rare, and some people stood up to get a better look, alarmed by the crimson face and the concave abdomen; a figure rushed down the stairs of the lecture hall to Rose's side, knocking over the student who'd begun to drone, imperturbable, through the first lines of his questionnaire, and leaned over to revive her while the eminent cardiologist dashed over in turn, aiming a pen-flashlight at her pupils. Rose frowned an eyebrow, opened one eye, then the other, and sat up energetically, peered at the crowd around her, and for the first time felt the pleasure of being applauded – she bowed flat-backed before the students in the bleachers, her first standing ovation.

The young man who had rushed over, furious to have been duped, reproached her for a lack of restraint in her performance, angina isn't a heart attack, you're getting the two mixed up, it's not the same thing, you should have played it with more delicacy and complexity, you're messing up the exercise. To make sure he's been understood, he lists the symptoms of angina one by one – constrictive chest pain, sensation of being crushed across the span of the chest, of being squeezed in a vice, sometimes with other characteristic pains in the lower jaw, one of the two forearms, or more rarely the back, the throat, but you don't collapse; then he details the symptoms of cardiac arrest – heartbeat shoots up to more than three hundred beats per minute, a ventricular fibrillation that causes the breath to stop, which causes a blackout, all in less than a minute – he keeps going, he could enumerate the treatments now, list the medications, the antiplatelet drugs that facilitate blood circulation and trinitrine that relieves pain by dilating the coronary arteries, he's bewitched, doesn't know what he's saying anymore, can't stop talking, tosses out sentences like lassos in order to keep her close to him, soon his heart races to an abnormally high speed, a tachycardia that approaches two hundred beats per minute, he's at risk of experiencing the very same ventricular fibrillation that he just described, at risk of fainting, ridiculous, Rose has turned toward him, slow, arrogant as a newborn star, looks him up and down and tells him all smiles that there was a bear sitting on her thorax, if he only knew, and says with a glint in her eye, sure, she'll start over again, as long as he plays the bear, he has the physique and the finesse, I'll tell you.

Virgilio Breva does indeed resemble a bear with his suppleness and slowness, his explosive energy. And yet he's a tall dark blond, stubbly beard and smooth hair tossed back, foaming at his nape, straight nose, fine features of a northern Italian (from Frioul). Otherwise the digitigrade gait of the sardana dancer when he's nearing a quintal, the corpulence of an ex-obese man calibrating him in thickness, in fullness, but without visible excrescence; in other words, without folds and without fat – his is simply a fleshy body, an even layer enwrapping him and growing fine toward the extremities of his arms, at his beautiful hands. An attractive and charismatic colossus, of a considerable stature that matches the eloquence of a warm voice, the enthusiastic though marked-by-excess moods, the bulimic appetite for knowledge and the exceptional capacity for hard work; yet his body has its painful fluctuations, an elasticity that causes him to suffer; it contains its share of shame and haunting – trauma from having been mocked, called chunky, tubby, roly-poly, or simply fat, anger for having been scorned, for having floundered sexually, mistrust of all kinds – and lodges all this self-disgust like a supplication in his stomach. Under constant scrutiny, he spent hours being examined for a speck of dust in his eye, was hydrated extensively for a sunburn, inspected closely for a hoarse voice, torticollis, fatigue: this body is Virgilio's great torment, his obsession, and his triumph – because now it pleases people, it's undeniable, you should see Rose's eyes roving over it – and those who are thick-skinned, jealous of his success, sneer and say that he became a doctor simply in order to learn to master this body, balance its moods, and tame its metabolism.

Top of the class at the residency in Paris, knocking back years of study rapidly, reducing them to twelve, university clinicat and assistantship of surgery included, while most students who chose the same course of study stretched it out over fifteen years – but I also don't have the means, he likes to say, charming, I'm not an old boy, and he plays up the role of the unknown wop, son of immigrants, illegitimate, the hardworking scholarship student, over the top – as creative with theory as he is prodigiously gifted in practice, flamboyant and proud, carried forward by an Atlantic ambition and an inexhaustible energy, he gets on a lot of nerves, it's true, and is often misunderstood – his mother, panicked by his success, valuing social above intellectual hierarchies, finally looks at him sideways, asks herself how did he do it, what was he made of, who did he think he was, this kid, while he flew into fits of rage to see her wringing her hands and then drying them on her apron, to hear her say plaintively on the day of his thesis defence that her presence was useless, that she wouldn't understand anything, that it wasn't her place, that she'd rather stay home and cook a feast just for him, these pâtés and these cakes that he loved.

He chose the heart, and then heart surgery. People were surprised, thinking he could have made a fortune examining naevi, injecting hyaluronic acid into frown lines and botox into the curves of cheekbones, reshaping the flabby stomachs of multiparous women, X-raying bodies, developing vaccines in Swiss laboratories, giving conferences in Israel and in the States about nosocomial infections, or becoming a high-end nutritionist. Or that he could have basked in glory by opting for neurosurgery, or even hepatic surgery, specialisations that sparkled in complexity and cutting-edge technology content. But no, he chose the heart. The good old heart. The state-of-the-art heart. The pump that squeaks, that leaks, that gets blocked, that's on the blink. A plumber's job, he likes to say: listen, poke and prod, identify the breakdown, change the parts, repair the machine – all that suits me perfectly, hamming it up, hopping from one foot to the other, he minimises the prestige of the discipline while at the same time allowing all of it to pander to his megalomania.

Virgilio chose the heart in order to exist at the highest level, counting on the organ's sovereign aura to rain glory down upon him, as it did upon the heart surgeons who whipped along hospital corridors, plumbers but also demigods. Because the heart exceeds the heart, he is well aware. Even dethroned – the muscle's movement no longer sufficient to separate the living from the dead – the heart, for Virgilio, is the body's central organ,the site of the most crucial and essential manifestations of life, and its symbolic stratification over centuries remains intact. And even more, as the cutting-edge mechanic and ultrapowerful fantasy operator all rolled into one, Virgilio sees the heart as the linchpin of depictions (paintings, etc.) that organise the relation of the human being to the body, to other beings, to Creation, and to the gods; the young surgeon is amazed at the way it's imprinted in language, at its recurrent presence precisely at this magic point of language, always situated at the exact intersection of the literal and the figurative, the muscle and the affect; he takes great delight in metaphors and figures of speech in which it is the analogy of life itself, and he repeats ad infinitum that although it was the first to appear, the heart will also be the last to disappear. One night at the Pitié, sitting in the staff room with the others in front of the huge fresco (painted by interns) – a spectacular entanglement of sexual scenes and surgical acts, a sort of gory orgy, campy and morbid, where a few bigwig faces appear from between enormous asses, breasts and pricks, among them one or two Harfangs, most often portrayed in the act, in obscene poses, doggy style or missionary, scalpel in hand – Virgilio told the story of the death of Joan of Arc with flair, eyes shining like marbles of obsidian, slowly recounting how the captive was brought in a cart from the prison to the Place du Vieux-Marché, the square where crowds had gathered; he described the slim figure in the tunic that had been doused with sulphur so she would burn faster, the pyre too high, the executioner Thérage who climbs up to tie her to the stake – Virgilio, galvanised by the attention of those listening, acts out the scene, tying solid knots in the air – before setting fire to the faggots like a man of experience, the arm that lowers the torch on to the coal and oily wood, the smoke lifting, the screams, Joan's cries before suffocation, and then the scaffolding blazing like a flare, and this heart they discovered intact after the body was burned, red beneath the embers, whole, so that they had to stoke the fire again to finally be rid of it.

Exceptional student, intern extraordinaire, Virgilio confounds the hospital hierarchy and struggles to nestle into groups with shared destinies, professing with equal militance an orthodox anarchism and a scorn for family dynasties, incestuous castes and biological collusions – and yet, like so many others, he is fascinated by all the Harfangs in the profession, drawn to these heirs, captivated by their reign, their health, their sheer numbers; he's curious about their properties, their tastes and their idioms, their humour and their clay tennis courts, so that being welcomed at their homes, sharing their culture, drinking their wine, complimenting their mothers, sleeping with their sisters – a crude devouring – all of this drives him crazy, and he schemes like a madman to get there, concentrating hard as a snake charmer, then hates himself as soon as he awakes, seeing himself in their sheets, suddenly uncouth, viciously offensive, an uncivilised bear rolling the bottle of Chivas under the bed, ransacking the porcelain from Limoges and the chintz curtains, and he always ends up fleeing from there, forlorn, lost.

His entry into the department of heart surgery at the Pitié-Salpêtrière raises his emotionalism a notch: conscious of his worth, he is immediately suspicious of barnyard rivalries, ignores docile dauphins, and works to get close to Harfang, to approach him intimately, to hear him think, doubt, tremble, to catch the very second of his decision and to perceive him in the momentum of his gesture; he knows that it's by being near him that he will learn from now on, here and nowhere else.

In the taxi Virgilio checks the composition of the Italian team on the screen of his *telefonino*, checks that Balotelli is playing, Motta too, yes, that's good, and Pirlo, and we have Buffon, then exchanges predictions and insults with two other clinic directors who'll go out tonight and drink to his health before a giant plasma screen, French men who detest the Italians' defensive game and cheer for a team that's under-prepared, physically. The vehicle speeds along the length of the Seine that lies flat and smooth as a lane, and as they near the entrance to the hospital, Chevaleret side, he makes an effort to quell his excitement and his torment. Soon he's simply smiling, not responding to the messages from the other two, forgetting about the bets and the one-upmanship. Rose's face reappears, he starts to type her a gallant text – something like: the curve of your eyes encircles my heart – and then changes his mind, the girl is nuts, she's crazy and dangerous, and he can let nothing, tonight, come to disturb his concentration, his self-control, he can let nothing affect the accomplishment of his work.

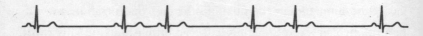

THE RETRIEVAL TEAMS ARRIVE ONE AFTER THE OTHER START-
ing at ten o'clock. The ones from Rouen show up in a car, since only
an hour's drive separates the CHU from the hospital in Le Havre,
while those from Lyon, Strasbourg and Paris will have taken a plane.

Coordinating teams have organised their transportation, called an
airline that accepted this Sunday mission, and made sure that the
little airport in Octeville-sur-Mer is open at night, formalising all the
logistical details. At the Pitié, Virgilio paws at the ground with impatience beside the nurse on duty who is phoning everyone – he doesn't
immediately notice the young woman in a white coat, also standing
there, silent, who pushes herself up from the wall when their gazes
meet and comes toward him, hello, I'm Alice Harfang, I'm the
new intern in the department, I'll be doing the retrieval with you.
Virgilio looks hard at her: no white lock grows in a cowlick in the
middle of her forehead but there is no doubt she is one of them, and
ugly, ageless, with yellow eyes and a nose like an eagle's beak, grand-
fathered in. A shadow comes over him. The handsome white coat
with the fur collar bothers him especially. Not exactly the perfect

190

outfit for slogging in hospitals. She's the kind of girl who rolls up like a tourist and believes money grows on trees, he thinks, irritated. Okay, well I hope at least you're not scared of flying? he asks curtly and then turns away as she replies no, not at all, the nurse on duty holding out a freshly printed map, you can go ahead, the plane is on the tarmac, take-off's in forty minutes. Virgilio picks up his bag and strides toward the department doors without a look at Alice, who follows close on his heels, then the lift, the taxi, the highways and the Bourget airport where they pass jetlagged businessmen in long cashmere overcoats clutching luxury holdalls, and soon they can both be seen climbing into a Beechcraft 200 and buckling their seat belts without having exchanged a single word.

The weather is fair: only a little wind and no snow, not yet. The pilot, a handsome woman in her thirties with perfectly straight teeth, announces good flying conditions and an estimated journey of forty-five minutes, then disappears into the cockpit. As soon as he is seated, Virgilio plunges into a financial magazine left behind on his seat; Alice turns toward the window and watches Paris become a tapestry of sparkling threads as the little plane gains altitude – the almond shape, the river and the islands, the squares and the main arteries, the bright zones of the boutique neighbourhoods, the dark zones of the projects, the parks, all of it darkening if you let your gaze wander from the heart toward the fringes of the capital, above the bright circle of the ring road; she follows the path of tiny red and yellow dots that flow along invisible streets, silent animation of the earth's crust. And then the Beechcraft rises above a hydrophilic substance and, here it is, the celestial night; and probably now, disconnected from Earth like this, projected outside any social cadastre, Virgilio begins to think of her differently, the woman who accompanies him – maybe he begins to find her less repellent – is this your first harvesting?

he asks. She starts, turns from the window and looks at him: yes, first harvesting, and first transplant. Virgilio closes his magazine and warns her: the first part of the night can be overwhelming, it's a multi-organ retrieval, the kid is nineteen, we'll probably take everything, the organs, the vessels, the tissues, shoop, we'll scrape out everything – his hand opens and closes in an ultra-rapid contraction of the fist. Alice looks at him – her expression, enigmatic, could just as easily signify "I'm scared" as "I'm a Harfang – did you forget already?" – then she brings her chairback up and fastens her seat belt again, as Virgilio, jostled, does the same: they're beginning the descent into Octeville.

The little airport has been opened specially for them, the runway is edged with status lights, the tower lit up at the top; the machine sets itself down, shaken by spasms, the door slides open and the foot-bridge unfolds, Alice and Virgilio step down on to the tarmac, and from that moment it's a single movement that carries them forward as though they were on a conveyor belt, a trajectory of a magical unbroken fluidity, crossing a barren exterior – this perimeter of pave-ment where you can hear the sea, a mobile and cosy interior – the taxi, an icy exterior – the hospital parking lot, and finally an interior where they know the codes – the surgical department.

Thomas Remige waits for them like the master of the house. Hand-shakes, coffees tossed back, they introduce themselves, connections are made and as always the name Harfang radiates its aura. Thomas lists those who are assembled: each team is a tandem composed of a senior surgeon and an intern, to which are added the anaesthetist, the nurse anaesthetist, the O.R. nurse, the nurse's aid, and himself, so thirteen of them altogether, it ends up being a lot of people inside, in the unassailable citadel, the secret cave accessible only to those who know the multiple pass codes, it's gonna be crammed in there, thinks Thomas.

The O.R. is ready. The scialytic projects a white light on to the operating table, vertical, casting no shadow – spots gathered into a circular cluster converge their rays on the body of Simon Limbeau that has just been brought in, in his bed, and it still has this air of animation – they are moved to see him like this. He's placed in the centre of the room – he is the heart of the world. A first circle around him demarcates a sterile zone that the circulating staff cannot cross: nothing can be touched, sullied, or infected, the organs they're preparing to collect here are sacred objects.

In a corner of the room, Cordelia Owl is apprehensive. She's changed her clothes, has left her mobile in a locker in the changing room, and the fact of being separated from it, no longer feeling the hard shape of the black case against her hip, vibratile and sly as a parasite, makes her shift into another reality, yes, it's here that it happens, she thinks, with her eyes riveted on the boy who is stretched out before her, and I'm here too. Trained in the O.R., she recognises the spaces but has never experienced anything but intense procedures aimed at saving patients, keeping them alive, and she struggles to grasp the reality of the operation that lies ahead, because the young man is already dead, isn't he, and the procedure is aimed at healing people other than him. She has prepared the materials, laid out the tools, and now quietly repeats to herself the order in which the organs are prepared, murmurs behind her mask: first, the kidneys; second, the liver; third, the lungs; and fourth, the heart; then she begins again, in reverse, recites to herself the steps of the harvesting established according to the length of ischemia the organ will tolerate – in other words, its survival time once blood flow is cut off: first, the heart; second, the lungs; third, the liver; and fourth, the kidneys.

The body is laid out, naked, arms outstretched in order to leave the ribcage and abdomen clear. It's prepared, shaved, swabbed. Then covered with a sterile surgical drape that marks out a window of skin, a cutaneous perimeter over the thorax and the abdomen.

Alright, we're ready to go. The first team present in the O.R., the urologists, gets the ball rolling – they are the ones who open the body, and they will be the ones to close it up again at the end. The two men bustle about, an odd pair, Laurel and Hardy, the long thin one is the surgeon and the short round one, the intern. It's the long thin one who leans over first and makes an incision – a laparotomy, so a kind of cross is drawn on the abdomen. The body is divided into two distinct areas at the level of the diaphragm: the abdominal area, holding the liver and kidneys, and the thoracic, holding the lungs and the heart. Next they place retractors at the edges of the incision, which are turned by hand to enlarge the opening – we can see that arm strength is called for, together with meticulous technical skill, and we suddenly glimpse the manual aspect of the operation, the physical confrontation with the reality of what is required here. The inside of the body, a murky and seeping interior, glows beneath the lamps.

The practitioners will prepare their organs one by one. Rapid and rigorous blades cut around each organ to free it from its attachments, ligaments, the various envelopes – but nothing is severed yet. The urologists, standing on either side of the table, talk during this sequence, the surgeon using the opportunity to train the intern; he leans over the kidneys, breaks down his movements and describes his technique while the student nods, asks the occasional question.

The Alsatians make their entrance an hour later, two women of the same height and corpulence; the surgeon, a rising star in the relatively select field of hepatic surgery, doesn't utter a single word, maintaining an impassive gaze behind little wire-rimmed glasses and working on her liver with a determination that resembles a battle, totally engaged in this action that seems to find its fullness through its very exertion, through practice, and her teammate doesn't let her eyes leave these hands for a second, hands of an unmatched dexterity.

Thirty-five more minutes pass and then the thoracic surgeons arrive. It's Virgilio's play now, his moment has come. He tells the Alsatians he's ready to make an incision, then cuts along the longitudinal section of the sternum. Unlike the others, he doesn't lean over – he keeps his back straight, head inclined, and arms held out in front of him – a way of keeping his distance from the body. The thorax is open and now Virgilio uncovers the heart, his heart, considers its volume, examines the ventricles, the atria, observes its beautiful contractile movement, and Alice watches him appreciating the organ. The heart is magnificent.

He proceeds with astounding rapidity, quarterback's arm and lace-maker's fingers, dissects the aorta and then, one by one, the venae cavae: he isolates the muscle. Alice, facing him on the other side of the operating table, is captivated by what she sees, by the procession around this body, by the sum of actions of which it is the object; she watches Virgilio's face, asks herself what it means for him to operate on a dead person, what he feels and what he's thinking and space suddenly pitches around her, as though in this place the separation between the living and the dead didn't exist anymore.

When the dissection is complete, they cannulate. The vessels are pierced with a needle in order to insert tiny tubes that inject a liquid to keep the organs cool. The anaesthetist monitors the donor's haemodynamic state on display screens, it's completely stable, while Cordelia furnishes the practitioners with the right tools, taking care to repeat the name of the compress, the number of the clamps or the blade at the moment when she places it in the hollow of the hand that's held out, open, in front of her, gloved in nitrile, and the more she distributes, the more sure her voice grows, the more she has the feeling of finding her place. It's ready now, the cannulation is done, they will be able to clamp the aorta – and all the practitioners in the O.R. identify what they have come to take on the anatomical cartography, pick out the piece that's intended for them.

Can we cross clamp? Virgilio's voice, loud in the room even though it's stifled by the mask, makes Thomas start. No, wait! He shouts it. All eyes turn toward him, hands go still above the body, arms at right angles, they suspend the operation as the coordinator weaves through to reach the bed and lean close to Simon Limbeau's ear. What he murmurs then, in his most human voice, even though he knows that his words sink into a lethal void, is the promised litany, the names of those who accompany him: he whispers that Sean and Marianne are with him, and Lou, too, and Grammy, he murmurs that Juliette is there – Juliette who knows, now, about Simon, a call from Sean around ten o'clock after she had left several messages on Marianne's mobile, each one more distraught, an incomprehensible call, because Simon's father seemed to be erring outside language, unable to formulate a single phrase anymore, only moans, chopped-up syllables, stuttered phonemes, choking sounds, and Juliette understood that there was nothing else to hear, that there were no words, that this was what she had to hear, and answered in a whisper I'm coming, then threw herself into the night, racing toward the Limbeaus' apartment, hurtling down the long hill, no coat, no scarf or anything, an elf in sneakers, keys in one hand, phone in the other, and soon the glassy cold became a burn, she consumed herself in the slope, dismantled figurine who nearly fell several times, she was trying so hard to co-ordinate her stride, and breathing poorly, not at all the way Simon had taught her to breathe, keeping no semblance of a regular rhythm and forgetting to exhale, the fronts of her tibias aching and her heels burning, her ears heavy as during an airplane landing, and stitches piercing her abdomen, she doubled over but kept running along the narrow pavement, scraping her elbow against the high stone wall that lined the curve, she hurtled down this same road that he had climbed for her five months earlier, the same turn in the opposite direction, that day of the *Ballade des pendus* and the lovers' capsule in red plastic that had lifted them up together, that day, that first day, she ran breathless now, and the cars that passed her as they drove up the hill slowed, catching her in the white rays of their headlights, the dumbstruck drivers continuing to watch her for a long time in their rear-view mirrors, a kid in a T-shirt in the street, at this hour, in this cold, and how panicked she looked! then she came into view of the bay window of the living room, dark, and ran even faster, entered the building, crossing a space barbed with flowerbeds and hedges that seemed to her like a hostile jungle, and she rushed again up the little stairway where she stumbled and fell, the carpet of leaves congealed by the cold forming a skating rink, she scratched her face, her temple and chin covered in mud, then the stairwell, three floors, and when she reached the landing, disfigured as the rest of them, unrecognisable, Sean opened the door before she even rang and took her in his arms, held her tightly, while behind him, in the dark, Marianne stood smoking in her coat near a sleeping Lou, oh Juliette, and then the tears came – then Thomas takes the headphones he has sterilised out of his pocket and puts them in Simon's ears, turns on the MP3 player, track seven, and the last wave forms on the horizon, it rises before the cliffs until it envelops the whole sky, forms and deforms, unfurling the chaos of matter and the perfection of the spiral in its metamorphosis, it scrapes the bottom of the ocean, stirs the sedimentary layers and shakes the alluvium, it uncovers fossils and tips over treasure chests, divulges these invertebrates that deepen the thickness of time, these hundred-and-fifty-million-year-old shelled ammonites and these beer bottles, these plane carcasses and these handguns, these bones whitened like bark, the sea floor as fascinating as a gigantic depository and an ultrasensitive membrane, a pure biology, it lifts the earth's skin, turns memory over, regenerates the ground where Simon Limbeau lived – the soft cleft of the dune where he shared a plate of fries and ketchup with Juliette, the pine forest where they took shelter during the squall and the bamboo thicket just behind, forty-metre stalks with their Asiatic sway; that day the warm drops perforated the grey sand and the smells mixed together, sharp and salty, Juliette's lips were grapefruit-coloured that time – until it finally explodes and scatters, the splashes fly about, it's a conflagration and a sparkling, while around the operating table the silence thickens, they wait, gazes meet above the body, toes shuffle, fingers wait it out, but each person allows for this pause at the moment of stopping Simon Limbeau's heart. At the end of the track, Thomas takes the headphones off and goes back to his place. Again: can we clamp?

– Clamp!

The heart stops beating. The body is slowly purged of its blood, which is replaced by a cooled liquid injected in a strong stream to rinse the organs from the inside, while ice cubes are immediately placed around them – and in that moment Virgilio probably casts a look at Alice Harfang to see if she's about to faint, because the blood that flows out of the body pours into a bin, and the plastic of the receptacle amplifies sounds like an echo chamber, it's really this sound more than the sight that makes an impression: but no, the young woman is there, perfectly stoic, although her forehead is pale and pearled with sweat, so he turns back to his work, the countdown has begun.

The thorax then becomes this site of ritual confrontation where heart surgeons and thoracic surgeons battle to gain a little more length in this stump of vein, or to gain a few extra millimetres of pulmonary artery – Virgilio, friendly but tense, finally fumes against the guy in front of him, think you could leave me a little slack, a centimetre or two, is that too much to ask?

Thomas Remige has slipped out of the O.R. to call the different departments where the transplants will take place so he can inform them of the time of the aortic clamping – 11.50 p.m. – a fact that immediately sharpens the timeline of the operation to come – preparation of the recipient, delivery of the organ, transplant. When he comes back, the first harvest is happening in total silence. Virgilio moves on to the ablation of the heart: the two venae cavae, the four pulmonary veins, the aorta and the pulmonary artery are severed – impeccable caesuras. The heart is explanted from Simon Limbeau's body. You can see it in the open air now, it's crazy, for a brief moment you can apprehend its mass and its volume, try to perceive its symmetrical form, its double bulge, its beautiful carmine or vermilion colour, try to see the universal pictogram of love, the emblem of the playing card, the T-shirt logo – I ♥ NY – the sculpted bas-relief from royal tombs and reliquaries, the symbol of Eros the charlatan, the portrayal of Jesus's sacred heart in devotional imagery – the organ held in hand and presented to the world, streaming tears of blood but haloed by a radiant light – or any emoticon indicating the infinite strata of sentimental emotions. Virgilio takes it and plunges it straightaway into a jar full of a translucent liquid, a cardioplegic solution that guarantees a temperature of four degrees Celsius – the organ must be cooled quickly in order to be conserved – and then this is protected in a sterile security pouch, then inside a second pouch, and the whole thing is buried in crushed ice inside a wheeled isothermal crate.

Once the crate is sealed, Virgilio says goodbyes all round, but none of those who encircle Simon Limbeau's body lift their heads, no one bats an eye, except the thoracic surgeon leaning over the lungs who answers in a loud voice you didn't leave me much leeway, eh, asshole, he lets out a staccato laugh, while the champion from Strasbourg prepares to uncover the fragile liver, concentrating like the gymnast before she mounts the beam – for a moment there you expected her to plunge her hands into a bowl of magnesium carbonate and rub her palms together – and while the urologists wait to claim the kidneys.

Alice lingers. She focuses on the scene, looks one by one at each of those who are gathered around the table and the inanimate body that is the stunning centre – Rembrandt's *The Anatomy Lesson* flashes before her eyes, she remembers that her father, an oncologist with long and twisted nails like talons, had hung a reproduction in the front hall, and often exclaimed as he tapped it with his index finger: there, *that* is the human being! but she was a dreamy child and preferred to see a council of witches rather than the doctors that made up her parentage; she would stand still for long moments before the strange characters admirably spread out around the cadaver, their clothes of a deep black, the immaculate ruffs on which their learnèd heads rested, the luxury of folds as precious as wafer origami, the lace trimmings and the delicate goatees, in the middle of which there was this pallid body, this mask of mystery, and the slit in the arm where you can see the bones and ligaments, the flesh into which the blade of the man in the black hat plunges, and more than admiring it, she *listened* to the painting, fascinated by the exchange there, and eventually she learned that piercing the peritoneal wall was considered for a long time to be a violation of the sacredness of the body of man, this creature of God, and understood that every form of knowledge contains its aspect of transgression, decided then to "do medicine", if it can even be said that she had a choice, because after all she was the eldest of four girls, the one her father brought with him to the hospital every Wednesday, the one to whom, on the day of her thirteenth birthday, he gave a professional stethoscope, whispering in her ear: the Harfangs are idiots, little Harfanguette, you'll fuck them all over, all of them.

Alice backs away, slowly, and all that she sees becomes fixed and illuminated, like a diorama. Suddenly, it's no longer an absolute matter that she perceives at the site of the body stretched out, a matter that can be used and that is shared out; it's no longer a stopped mechanism that they dissect in order to keep the best parts – it becomes instead a substance of an incredible potentiality: a human body, its power and its end, its human end – and it's this emotion, more than any fountain of blood poured out into a plastic bin, that can finally make her look away. Virgilio's voice is already far away behind her, you coming? What are you doing? Come on! She turns and runs to catch up to him in the corridor.

A specialised vehicle drives them back to the airport. They streak along the surface of the earth, and their eyes accompany the movement of the numbers on the dashboard clock, follow the dancing bars of light that lie down and stand up again, come and go in place of needles on their watches, show up as pixelated shapes on their telephone screens. Then a call, Virgilio's cell lights up. It's Harfang. How is it?

– It's mint.

They skirt the city to the north and take the road for Fontaine-la-Mallet, passing shapes that are at once compact and imprecise, border neighbourhoods, ghettos planted in the fields behind the city, swarms of suburban houses divided into plots around a ring of pavement, crossing through a forest, still no stars, no flash of an airplane or a flying saucer, nothing, the driver blasts along the service road well above the speed limit, he's an experienced driver, used to this type of mission, he looks straight ahead, forearms still and tense, and murmurs into a minuscule microphone linked to the latest earpiece, I'm coming, don't fall asleep, I'm coming. The crate is wedged into the trunk and Alice visualises the different hermetic cases that encapsulate the heart, these membranes that protect it, she imagines that it is the motor propelling them through space, like the reactor of a rocket. She turns and lifts one hip to peer over the seat back, makes out the sticker on the side of the crate in the dark, and deciphers, among the information necessary for the traceability of the organ, a strange note: Element or Product of the Human Body for Therapeutic Use. And just below, the donor's Cristal number.

Virgilio leans his head back against the seat, exhales, his eyes drift over Alice's profile, shadow puppet against the window, he's suddenly unsettled by her presence, softens: you okay? The question is unexpected – a guy who's been so unpleasant up until now – the radio propagates Macy Gray's voice singing *shake your booty, boys and girls, there is beauty in the world* in a loop, and Alice suddenly wants to cry – an emotion that seizes her from inside, lifts and sways her back and forth – but holds back her tears and grits her teeth as she turns her head: yeah, yeah, I'm great. He pulls his phone out of his pocket then for the umpteenth time, but instead of checking the time, drums on the buttons, growing increasingly aggravated, it's not loading, he mutters, damn, damn. Alice, emboldened, asks him, something wrong? Virgilio doesn't lift his head to answer her, it's the game, I wanted the score for the game, and without turning his head the driver says coldly it's Italy, 1–0. Virgilio lets out a whoop, makes a fist that he lifts inside the car, then immediately asks: who scored? The guy puts his indicator on and brakes, a bright intersection lays out a whitish gap before them: Pirlo. Bemused, Alice watches Virgilio rapidly composing one or two victory texts as he murmurs, that's great, then he lifts an eyebrow in her direction, fantastic player that Pirlo! his smile overwhelms his face, and here already is the airport, the roar of the sea right there at the bottom of the cliff, and the crate they roll along the tarmac to the steps and hoist into the cabin, this matryoshka crate that holds the transparent plastic security bag that holds the container that holds the special jar that holds Simon Limbeau's heart – that holds nothing less than life itself – the potential for life, and that, five minutes later, flies off into the air.

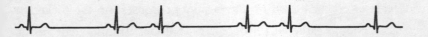

MARIANNE DOESN'T SLEEP, AS YOU MIGHT SUSPECT, DOESN'T close her eyes or doze for even a second – pain smashes her open, and she sinks into an altered state, that's where she can withstand. At 11.50 we see her sit straight upright all of a sudden on the living room couch – could it be that she feels the moment when the blood stops flowing in the aorta? Could it be that she has an intuitive sense of this moment? Despite the kilometres that stretch out along the estuary, between the apartment and the hospital, could there be an impalpable proximity that gives the night a fantastic mental depth, vaguely terrifying, as though magnetic lineaments hurtle through a spatio-temporal rift and connect her to this restricted space where her child is, weaving a zone of wakefulness.

Polar night – it seems as if the opaque sky is dissolving, the layer of clouds tearing open, woolly, and the Big Dipper appears. Simon's heart is migrating now, it's speeding over the orbs, along the rails, along the roads, moving inside this crate whose slightly nubby plastic walls shine in beams of electric light, escorted with an unmatched attention, the same way they escorted princes' hearts in olden times, the way they escorted their entrails and their skeletons, the body divided up to be distributed, inhumed in a basilica, a cathedral, an abbey, in order to guarantee an entitlement to his lineage, prayers for his salvation, a future for his memory – you could hear the sounds of hooves from the furrow of roads, on the clay of the villages and cobblestones of the cities, their slow and sovereign steps, and then you could make out the flames from torches that cast liquid shadows on the leaves, on the facades of houses, on the flickering faces, people gathered on doorsteps, napkins around their necks, they stepped out and made signs to each other in silence as they watched the extraordinary cortège pass by, the black coach drawn by six horses in full mourning attire, caparisoned with precious drapes and surplices, the escort of twelve riders in long black coats and veils carrying torches, and sometimes also pages and valets on foot, brandishing white wax votives, sometimes also Gardes du Corps, and the rider in tears who leads all of them is the one to accompany the heart to its tomb, progressing toward the depths of the crypts, toward the chapel of a selected monastery or a native castle, toward a niche carved into black marble and flanked by twisted columns, a shrine topped with a radiant crown, decorated with precious insignia and coats of arms, Latin mottoes deployed on banners of stone, and often they tried to catch a glimpse inside the coach through the slit in the curtains, to the bench where the official in charge of the sacred transaction sat – the one who would place the heart into the rightful hands of those who would watch over it and pray for it, most often a confessor, a friend, or a brother – but the darkness never allowed them to see this man, nor the reliquary placed on a cushion of black taffeta, and even less the heart inside, the *membrum principalissimum*, the king of the body, placed in the centre of the chest like the sovereign in his realm, like the sun in the sky, this heart nestled in gauze with gold brocade, this heart they lamented.

Simon's heart migrated toward another part of the country; his kidneys, his liver and his lungs reached other provinces, they rushed toward other bodies. In all this splintering, what would remain of the wholeness of her son? How to connect his singular memory to this diffracted body? What would be left of his presence, of his light in the world, of his ghost? These questions whirl around her like scalding hoops and then Simon's face forms before her eyes, intact and irreducible – it's him. She feels a deep sense of calm. The night burns outside like a gypsum crystal desert.

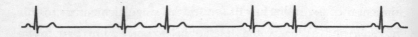

AT THE PITIÉ, THEY ENCIRCLE CLAIRE. SHE'S WHEELED INTO another room in the heart surgery department that will have been completely scoured, disinfected; a glazing of transparency covers the surfaces, effluvia of detergent hovers in the room. A movable bed that's too high, a blue leatherette armchair, a barren table, and, in a corner of the room, a bathroom door, half-open. She puts her bag down and sits on the bed. She's dressed all in black – this old sweater split at the shoulders – and her form is cut out perfectly in the room, like a sketch. Texts begin to come in on her phone, her sons, her mother, her best friend, they're all on their way, they're racing to get there, but no message from the man with the foxgloves who has just rested on his heels against a bamboo hedge among stray dogs and wild pigs in a village on the Gulf of Siam.

The nurse who comes in says chummily, hands on her hips: so, it's your big night! She's crowned with a helmet of salt-and-pepper hair and wears square-framed glasses; a light rosacea colours her cheekbones. Claire lifts her palms toward the sky and shrugs her shoulders, smiles, yes, tonight the sky's the limit! The nurse holds out flat trans-

208

parent sachets that shimmer beneath the overhead lights like glass noodles, leans forward, a pendant comes unstuck from her skin, brief twinkling in the void – it's a little silver heart engraved with a promise, *today more than yesterday and less than tomorrow*, little jewel listed in mail-order catalogues; Claire follows its sway with her eyes, captivated – then the nurse straightens up, points to the sachets: these are the clothes for the O.R., you'll put them on to go there, and Claire looks at them with this mix of impatience and reluctance that is the very fabric of the feeling that has been plaguing her for more than a year now, and the other name for waiting. She answers, feigning composure, but we'll wait for the heart to arrive first, right? The woman shakes her head and looks at her watch, no, you're heading to the O.R. in about two hours, as soon as we've received the results of your checkup; the heart will arrive at about half past midnight, you'll need to be ready, the transplant will happen right after. She leaves the room.

Claire unpacks her things, places her toiletries in the bathroom, plugs in her phone charger, puts the phone on her bed; she personalises the place. Calls her sons – they're running on the pavement, down the hallways of the Metro, she hears the echo of their steps in the corridors, we're on our way, we're coming, they pant in distress. They want to reassure her, to support her. They are mistaken: she's not scared of the operation. It's not that. What torments her is the idea of this new heart, and that someone had to die today in order for all of this to happen, and that he or she could invade and transform her, change her – stories of grafts, cuttings, fauna and flora.

She turns in circles in the room. If this is a gift, it's certainly a strange kind, she thinks. There's no giver in this exchange, no one intended to give a gift here, and likewise there is no recipient, because she doesn't have the choice of refusing the organ, she has to receive it if she wants to survive, so what then, what is it? The release back into circulation of an organ that's still usable, carrying out its job as a pump? She starts undressing, sits on the bed, pulls off her boots, her socks. The meaning of this transfer that she has the luck to receive through unbelievable chance – the amazing compatibility of her blood and genetic code with those of a being who died today – all of this goes hazy, out of focus. She doesn't like this idea of undue privilege, of a lottery, feels like the stuffed animal grabbed by the claw from the jumble of thingamajigs heaped up behind glass at the fairground. And above all, she will never be able to say thank you – and that's just it. It's technically impossible – thank you, these radiant words whispered into the void. She will never be able to show any form of gratitude toward the donor and his family, or make a reciprocal gift in order to free herself from the infinite debt, and she's shot through with the idea that she will be ensnared forever. The ground is frozen beneath her feet, she's scared, everything retracts.

She goes to the window. Figures hurry along the paths to the hospital, slow cars circulate between buildings that draw the anatomical map of the human body in the night, organ by organ, pathology by pathology, separating children from adults, grouping together mothers, the elderly, the dying. She would like to be able to kiss her sons before putting on this paper chasuble that floats without covering her and gives her the feeling of being naked in a gust of air, keeps her eyes dry but struggles to break down the enormity of all that's happening, and her in the midst of it, places her hand there, between her breasts, feels its rhythm, always a little too fast despite the medication, always a little unpredictable too, and says its name out loud: heart.

*

Even after hours of interviews with the doctors in charge of her psychological evaluation when the transplant was first proposed – assessment of her emotional attachments, measure of her degree of social integration, survey of her comportment in the face of fatigue and anxiety, of her willingness to face post-op treatments that would be difficult and long – no one could tell her what would happen to her heart, afterwards. Maybe somewhere there's a junkyard for organs, she says to herself, taking off her jewellery and her watch, a landfill of sorts, and hers will be tossed there with the others, carried away from the hospital through the service doors in big garbage bags; she envisions a container for organic matter where her heart will be recycled, returned to a indistinct matter, compost of remodelled flesh that the boundlessly cruel Atrides would serve to their famished rivals in the palace dining room, galette or steak tartar, feed given to the dogs in large dishes, bait for bears and marine mammals -- and maybe these creatures would be transformed after ingesting the substance, their scaly skin sprouting platinum hair like her own, maybe they would grow long velvety eyelashes.

A knock and then he enters the room directly without waiting for a reply, it's Emmanuel Harfang. He plants himself before her, says the heart will be harvested around eleven o'clock, the organ's specs are impeccable, then he grows quiet, observes her: you wanted to talk to me. She sits on the bed, rounds her back, places her hands flat on the mattress and crosses her ankles, her feet are ravishing, her nails are painted bright purple, they explode in the chlorotic room like foxglove petals, yes, I have some questions, questions about the donor, Harfang shakes his head as though he thinks she's pushing it, she knows the answer. We've already talked about this. But Claire insists, her blonde hair forming hooks against her cheeks, I want to be able to think about the person. She adds, persuasive: for example, where will this heart be coming from, if it's not from Paris? Harfang stares at her, frowns, how does she even know that much? then consents: Seine-Maritime. Claire closes her eyes, accelerates: male or female? Harfang, tit for tat, male; he heads for the door that's open on to the corridor, she hears him heading off, opens her lids again, wait, his age, please. But Harfang has already gone.

Her three sons arrive together just after, looking awful; the oldest, terribly anxious, won't let go her hand, the second whirls about the room and repeats over and over everything's going to be fine, the youngest has brought a pack of heart-shaped candies. Harfang's an ace, the best in his field, seventy heart transplants a year, and the best team, you're in good hands, he tells her in a small, trembling voice. She nods mechanically, observes his face without really listening, I know, don't worry. It's harder with her mother who can't stop snivelling that life is unfair, that she wants to take her place under the knife – saying it's more natural, more conceivable, that she be the one to die, or at least the one to risk her life first – Claire grows impatient, but I'm not going to die, I have no intention of dying – and the boys, incensed, speak sharply to their grandmother, that's enough! they're all foundering here. The nurse comes back to the room, taps her watch face, and hurries things along, everything is in order, you need to get ready now. Claire kisses her sons, caresses their cheeks, murmurs to each of them, see you tomorrow, my love.

Later, naked, she steps into the shower and washes herself for a long time with Betadine, spraying her entire body with yellow liquid, and

212

rubbing herself vigorously. When she's dry, she pulls on the sterile tunic, and then begins to wait again.

Around ten o'clock, the anaesthetist comes into the room, is everything alright? She's a tall woman, narrow shoulders and hips, a swan's neck, pale smile, she has long cold hands that brush Claire's own when she holds out a first dose of medication – to relax you – and Claire lies back on the bed, suddenly worn out even though she's wound up like never before. An hour later, the O.R. porter comes in, takes hold of the handles on her bed, they'll operate on you on the table and bring you back to your bed afterwards, and then he transfers her without a word. They travel along metres and metres of corridors, she doesn't know where to rest her eyes, sees the dull ceilings file past, and sinuous electrical wires like river serpents. Her heart accelerates bit by bit as they reach the O.R., pass through airlocks and coded double doors. The space becomes further isolated, then she is brought into a small room where she's told to wait. They'll come get you. Time dilutes, nearly midnight.

Behind the door to the O.R., the anaesthetist checks the equipment set-up for the patient's monitoring: places electrodes for cardiac monitoring, inserts arterial catheter lines for continuous blood pressure monitoring, and this apparatus that pinches the end of the finger to monitor oxygenation of the blood. She administers the intravenous, hangs the pouch of translucent liquid, checks the seals – simple gestures, modelled on thirty years' experience, perfectly executed – okay, we're good to go, is everyone here? But everyone isn't quite here, the team is getting ready in the change room, pulling on sky-blue pyjamas, short-sleeved shirts and long-sleeved jackets, each one puts on at least two plastic caps to be sure to cover the entire scalp, and two masks over their mouths. Slippers, overslippers, sterile gloves in multiple pairs that will be changed several times over.

Thorough washing in plenty of water, forearms soaped up to the elbows with disinfectant, nails cleaned, once, twice, three times. Then they head into the O.R. Indistinct bodies take their places, check the machines, but although the faces have disappeared, the aura, the size, the way of moving, the corpulence, the body language and the eyes remain to form another language within this enclosure. Present are a perfusionist, an O.R. intern, two dressing nurses specialised in packing the organs, and two anaesthesiologists – Harfang's been working with this pair of old girlfriends for thirty years; he did his first transplant with them.

And here he is now, looking as if he's just set off on a race. He's put on a high-coverage surgical gown that slips on from the front and is knotted at the back, one sleeve attached to the thumb by a ring – its half-calf length is reminiscent of butcher's aprons that narrow the hips. He comes over to Claire for a last word: the heart will be here in thirty minutes, it's gorgeous, it was made for you, the two of you will get along just fine. Claire smiles: but you'll wait until it's in the O.R. before taking this one out, right? Harfang, taken aback: are you serious?

Claire is anaesthetised. Images begin to appear behind her eyelids, plastic gush of soft shapes and warm tones, infinite metamorphosis of surfaces, kaleidoscopic spreading of cells and fibres as the nurses make her head and body disappear beneath large sheets of yellow plastic, covered in turn with sterile surgical drapes: only a small perimeter of skin remains visible, pale beneath the lamp beams, poignant, this area they're going to carve into. Harfang makes the first gestures, he inscribes the line of the incisions to come on her thorax with a sterile pencil, takes note of the precise places for small openings – tubes carrying a system of cameras will be slid inside the body. Then the anaesthetist, glued to the O.R. telephone, turns and says: okay, they're on their way.

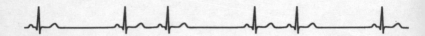

ANOTHER OPERATING ROOM IN A NOCTURNAL ESTUARY, BUT THIS one empty, the order of departure of the teams inverse to the order of organs recovered, the last ones to lean over Simon Limbeau are those who retrieve the kidneys, the urologists, they're always the last. And they are the ones responsible for restoring the body, for making it look whole again.

Thomas Remige is there too, face shining with fatigue, cheeks flat, and even though these are different hours that are beginning – flaring out as they near the end of the process, hours delayed in a timeline that is at once slower and of a softer texture – his presence grows sharper, more intense. Each one of his actions, even the most imperceptible, expresses the idea that no, it's not over, no, it's not over yet. Of course he exasperates the others as he cranes his neck over their shoulders, as he anticipates the movements of the surgeons and the nurses. It would be so easy to let go a little now, to let a point or two slide, to expedite the final procedures, to close out the thing, in the end what would it change? Thomas silently resists, countercurrent to the general exhaustion or the urgency to close up shop, he lets nothing slide: this phase of the retrieval, the restoration of the donor's body, cannot be trivialised, it's a mending: they have to mend, now, mend the damage. Put that which was given back together, the way it was given. Otherwise, it's just savagery. Around him, eyes roll, people sigh: don't worry, what do you expect, we won't botch anything, everything will be done as it should be.

Simon Limbeau's body is hollow, the skin appears to have been suctioned out from the inside in places. It didn't have this atrophied appearance when it entered the O.R., it screams mutilations endured, it's a violation of the promise made to the parents. They have to fill it. The practitioners quickly make a lining using surgical pads and compresses, crude stuffing that they must model as best they can to correspond to the volume and shape of the organs that have been recovered, then position them inside. Hands busy themselves and the actions performed are those of a restoration: it's a matter of giving Simon Limbeau back his original appearance, so that it's him, and this image of him, that may be archived in the memory of those who will see him tomorrow at the funeral home, so they might recognise him as the person he was.

They are closing up the body now – over its emptiness, its silence. The running stitch suture – sewn with a single thread, knotted at each end – will be delicate, careful, the needle of the practitioner, fine and precise, tracing a straight dotted line, and what's striking is that the act of sewing, this archaic gesture sedimented in human memory since the eyed needles of Paleolithic times, could reach the operating room and be the conclusion to an operation of such technological advancement. Also, the surgeon works with absolute intuition, totally unconscious of his movements, his hand carrying out regular loops above the wound, short and identical loops that will lace up and close the skin. Before him, the young intern continues to observe and learn

– it's the first time he, too, is present at a multiple-organ retrieval and he probably would have liked to do the suture himself, probably would have liked to bring his hand, too, to the donor's body in order to join the collective gesture, but the density of the operation has saturated his perceptions, and black butterflies of fatigue or nervousness flutter in his field of vision, he stiffens, tells himself he didn't flinch when the blood poured out into the pail, at least that's something, and that the main thing is to stay standing until the very end.

At one-thirty, the urologists put down their tools, lift their heads, exhale, pull down their masks, and leave the O.R.; they take the kidneys with them. The only ones remaining are Thomas Remige and Cordelia Owl, who seems to stay standing under the effect of a residual tension, she hasn't slept for nearly forty hours and she has the feeling that if she stops even for a second, she'll fall over, collapse on the spot. She begins the work of the end. Takes an inventory of the instruments, fills out the labels, notes numbers on printed sheets, writes down the hours, and these administrative formalities, carried out with the rigour of an automaton, leave her mind free to ramble, for flashes to blaze in her brain, cross-fades linking fragments of bodies, snippets of words, portions of places – the hospital corridor opens on to an alleyway of exquisite stenches, the lock of hair trembles above the lighter flame, the orange streetlamps undulate vertically in the eyes of her lover, the sirens with green hair stir on the body of a van, her phone finally vibrates in the night – porous continuum on to which Simon Limbeau's face is etched, the one she cleaned this afternoon, that she examined and caressed, and this young woman, body sprinkled with brown hickeys – a panther's skin – thinks suddenly of the time it will take for these hours to decant, for her to be able to filter out the violence, clarify the meaning – what did I just live through? Her eyes mist over, she looks at her watch, lowers her mask, I have to go back up to the department in a minute, the intern is alone upstairs, I'll be back. Thomas nods without looking up, it's fine, I'll finish up, take your time. The girl's steps recede and the door of the O.R. closes behind her. Thomas is alone now. He scans the place with a slow circular sweep of his eyes and what he sees makes him shudder: the place has been laid to ruin, chaos of material and electrical wires, displaced screens, used tools, sullied cloths piled up on work tables, the operating table soiled and the ground splashed with blood. Anyone who stuck a head in would blink their eyes against the cold light and then form an image of a battleground after the onslaught, an image of war and violence – Thomas shivers, and gets to work.

Simon Limbeau's body has become a corpse. What life leaves behind when it has slipped away, what death leaves on the battlefield. It's a violated body. Frame, carcass, hide. The boy's skin slowly turns the colour of ivory, it seems to harden, haloed in this raw light that falls from the scialytic lamp, it seems to become a dry carapace, a breastplate, a suit of armour, and the scars across the abdomen are reminiscent of a mortal blow – the lance in Christ's side, the sword strike of the warrior, the knight's blade. And whether it's this act of sewing that recreates the bard's song, the one of the rhapsody of Ancient Greece, whether it's Simon's face, the beauty of this young man risen from the ocean wave, his hair still full of salt and curled like the manes of Ulysses' companions, whether it's this that unsettles him, or his scar in the shape of a cross, Thomas begins to sing. A fine song, barely audible to he or she who might find themselves in the same room with him, but a song that synchronises with the actions that make up the last offices for the dead, a song that accompanies and describes, a song for the deposition.

The necessary material for preparing the body before it's taken to the morgue is laid out on a crash cart. Thomas has pulled a disposable apron on over his shirt, pulled on single-use gloves, gathered towels – they too are single use, one time only, for Simon Limbeau – and soft cellulose compresses, a yellow garbage bag. He begins by closing the boy's eyes using a dry eye pad, and then, to close his mouth, he rolls two pieces of cloth, places one beneath the occiput so as to flex the neck, while the other supports the chin, pressing vertically against the thorax. Next, he removes everything that invades the body, threads and tubes, drips and catheter, he takes out everything that criss-crosses it, enlaces it, obstructs the view of it – he frees it and then Simon Limbeau's body appears in the light, suddenly more naked than naked: human body catapulted outside humanity, troubling matter drifting in the magmatic night, in the unshaped space of non-sense, but an entity to which Thomas's song confers a presence, a new meaning. Because this body that life has shattered becomes whole again beneath the hand that washes it, in the breath of the voice that sings; this body that has undergone something extraordinary now becomes part of the greater death, the company of others. It becomes the subject of praises, it is embellished.

Thomas washes the body, his movements are calm and loose, and his voice draws upon the corpse so as not to falter, just as it dissociates from language in order to grow strong, frees itself from earthly syntax to reach that exact place in the cosmos where life and death meet: it breathes in and breathes out, breathes in and breathes out; it escorts the hand that revisits the contours of the body one last time, recognising each fold and each span of skin, including the tattoo across the shoulder, this emerald black arabesque inscribed in his skin the summer he told himself his body was his own, that his body expressed something essential about him. Thomas applies pressure now to the puncture points where tubes have pierced the epidermis, and dresses the boy in a change of clothes – he even arranges his hair so that his face becomes radiant. The song grows louder still in the operating room as Thomas wraps the body in an immaculate sheet – this sheet that will be knotted at the head and the feet – and watching him work, funerary rituals come to mind, ones that conserve the beauty of the Greek hero come to die with intention on the battlefield, these rituals created to restore his image, to guarantee him a place in human memory. So that societies, families, and poets will be able to sing his name, commemorate his life. It's a good death, it's the song of a good death. Not an elevation, the sacrificial offertory, not an exaltation of the soul that clouds in ascending circles toward Heaven, but an edification: this song reconstructs the singularity of Simon Limbeau. It causes the young man to rise up from the dune, surfboard under his arm, run along the shore with others beside him, it makes him fight over some insult, hopping from foot to foot with fists up by his face and elbows in tight, it makes him thrash and jump in the mosh pit at a concert, wild, and sleep on his stomach in the bed he's had since he was a child, it makes him spin Lou around – little ankles fluttering above the kitchen floor – it makes him sit down at midnight with his mother who's smoking in the kitchen, to talk about his father, it makes him undress Juliette, and hold out his hand so she can jump down from the seawall, it propels him into a post-mortem space where death doesn't reach, a space of immortal glory, of mythography, of song and literature.

*

Cordelia reappears an hour later. She's made the rounds of the department, she's pushed open the doors, has looked in on those in the recovery room, she's checked the vitals in the private rooms, the flow of electric syringes and diuresis, she's leaned over the beings that sleep there, over their faces that sometimes twist in suffering, she's observed their positions, listened to their breath, and now she goes back to see Thomas. She catches him singing, hears him even before she sees him because his voice has grown strong now, and she freezes, deeply moved. With her back flat against the door to the O.R., hands at her sides, head thrown back, she listens.

Later, Thomas lifts his eyes. Good timing. Cordelia approaches the table. The white sheet covers Simon up to his neck, throwing his facial features into relief, the grain of his skin, the transparency of cartilage, and the flesh of his lips. Does he look handsome? Thomas asks her; yes, very, she answers. And then their eyes meet, deliberate, full, and they lift the body together, which, in spite of everything, is still heavy, standing at either extremity to slide him on to a stretcher, in a shroud, before calling the funeral home. Tomorrow morning, Simon Limbeau will be brought back to his family, to Sean and Marianne, to Juliette and Lou, to the people close to him, he will be given back *ad integrum*.

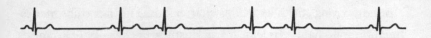

THE PLANE LANDS IN BOURGET AT 12.50 A.M. TIME SHARPENS.
A car is waiting for them, impeccable logistical coordination. This is
no taxi, but a specialised car for just this type of mission, thermally
regulated – the inscription on the doors says: priority vehicle, organ
transplant. A profound calm reigns inside the car: although the tension is palpable, there is no hint of a staged emergency scene, a
re-enactment for a televised report on the glory of transplants and
the heroic human chain, no hysterical pantomime with a red stop-
watch running in the corner of the screen, no blue lights or motorcycle
squadron with white helmets and black boots leading the way, armada
of stiff thumbs and impassive faces, contracted jaw muscles. The process unfolds in a controlled manner and traffic on the highway is clear
for the moment, the flow of weekend return trips this Sunday evening
has already been diluted: before them Paris rises beneath a dome of
corpuscular light A call from the O.R. when they're passing Garonor:
the patient is here, we'll begin preparations, where are you? We're ten
minutes from La Chapelle. We're on time, Virgilio murmurs, and
looks at Alice, her profile of a night bird – the concave of her forehead,
her beak-like nose, her beautiful silky skin – alights on the fur collar
of her white coat, she sure does have a Harfang face, he thinks.

Outside the Stade de France, they hit a traffic jam. Shit. Virgilio sits up straight, immediately tense. What the hell are they still doing here? The driver doesn't blink. It's the game, they don't want to go home. The bottleneck is made up of cars full of young guys drunk on celebration leaning out the windows in the cold, prancing the Italian flag around on long sticks, as well as charter buses for fan clubs, not to mention long-haul refrigerator trucks stuck in the euphoric tangle. They're signalling a pile-up ahead. Alice lets out a cry, Virgilio grows even more tense. Centimetre by centimetre, the driver manages to widen the gaps between cars to slip his vehicle through and reach the emergency lane where he drives at a reduced speed for nearly a kilometre, passing the nodal accident, after which the lane is empty and acceleration powerful, reflectors spaced out along the guard rail becoming no more than a long luminous ribbon in the night. Congestion again at La Chapelle. We'll take the ring road. The points of entry are strung out along the city's borderline to the east, from Aubervillier to Bercy, long curve at the end of which the vehicle nudges back over to the right, enters the city, and then there are the banks of the Seine, the towers of the library, a turn to the left and they drive up Vincent-Auriol boulevard, stop at Chevaleret, enter the hospital grounds, it's here, the vehicle stops in front of the buildings – thirty-two minutes, not bad – Virgilio smiles.

In the O.R., the others barely lift their heads when they show up, bringing the treasure to the foot of the bed together like a trophy to the feet of the master. Their arrival scarcely creates a stir, because the operation, here, has already begun. The team is already wearing sterile clothing, arms washed, hands disinfected – and now the only thing that Virgilio sees of Alice are her strange eyes, slow and condensed, where scattered yellows coagulate, chartreuse and honey, smoky topaz. Harfang, though, does finally toss out: so, everything went okay with the heart? And Virgilio, in the same relaxed tone, says: yes, just a pile-up on the way back into town.

The heart is placed in a basin, close to the bed. Alice climbs on to a small standing stool at the end of the table, she will observe the transplant; her legs wobble a little as she pulls herself up the step, while Virgilio comes forward to take his place as O.R. intern, just managing to hold back from taking the instruments in his own hand. Everything in him is expressing his desire to be there, beneath the three scialytic lights above the thorax, and to be there across from Harfang. They're working together, now.

Suddenly, as he reveals Claire's heart, Harfang whistles and exclaims that this one isn't in the best shape, it might be time to find a new one, and around him they agree, half-laughing – it's surprising to find out that he's a bit of a crowd-pleaser in the O.R., putting on a show, while also keeping each of his team members under formidable pressure, seeing everything, even what's happening behind him. But the O.R. is truly the only place where he feels himself existing, where he's able to express who he is, his atavistic passion for his work, his maniacal rigour, his faith in human beings, his megalomania, his dreams of power; it's here that he convokes his lineage and remembers one by one those who developed the act of transplanting, scientifically – the first to perform one, the pioneers, Christiaan Barnard in the Cape in 1967, Norman Shumway at Stanford in 1968, and Christian Cabrol here, at the Pitié, men who had invented the transplant, had conceived of it mentally, had composed and decomposed the process hundreds of times before carrying it out, all men from the 1960s, workaholics, charismatic stars, media-friendly competitors who argued over who would do the first operations and didn't hesitate to steal from one another, playboys of multiple marriages surrounded by girls in mod boots and Mary Quant miniskirts made up like Twiggy, autocrats of a mad audacity, guys covered with accolades but still hungry for success.

First they have to work on the vessels that carry the blood in and out of the organ. One by one, the veins are cut, closed, manipulated – Harfang and Virgilio work fast, but it seems that the speed is what carries the action, that if their hands slowed they would risk trembling – then, it's impressive, the heart is lifted from the body and the extracorporeal circulation is put in place: a machine replaces Claire's heart for two hours, a machine that will reproduce the blood circuit in her body. At that moment, Harfang requests silence – he clinks a blade against a metal tube and then, from behind his mask, recites the ritual phrase for this stage of the operation: *Exercitatio Anatomica de Motu Cordis et Sanguinis in Animalibus* (An Anatomical Exercise on the Motion of the Heart and Blood in Living Beings) – homage to William Harvey, the first physician to describe, in 1628, the human circulatory system in its entirety, and who had already named the heart as a pump with a hydraulic effect, a muscle ensuring the continuity of the flow by its movements and pulsations. Without missing a beat, each person in the O.R. responds: amen!

The perfusionist is disconcerted by this strange ritual. He doesn't know Latin and wonders what's going on. He's a nurse with turned-up eyelashes, a young guy, twenty-five or twenty-six, the only one here who has never worked with Harfang before. He's sitting on a high stool in front of his machine, rather like a disc-jockey at the turntable, and no one here would know better than him how to find their way around the pandemonium of wires that protrude from big black boxes. Filtered, oxygenated, the blood rushes into a tangle of thin transparent tubes, colour-coded stickers identifying the direction of flow. On the screen, the electrocardiogram is flat, the body temperature is thirty-two degrees Celsius, but Claire is fully alive. The anaesthetists take turns checking the vitals and administration of the I.V.s. We can go ahead.

Virgilio bends down to pick up the heart from the container. The ligatures of the different pockets that protect it are sprayed with disinfectant, then opened, and finally he takes the organ from the jar, holds it with both hands, and places it deep inside the ribcage. Alice, still poised on tiptoe on the metal stool, keeps her eyes fixed on it, fascinated, and nearly loses her balance when she leans forward to see what's happening there, inside the body; she's not the only one to crane her neck like that – the O.R. intern who's come to stand beside Harfang leans forward too, so dripping with sweat that his glasses slide down his nose and he nearly loses them – he pulls back at the very last moment to push them up his nose and bumps into a drip, watch it, please, the anaesthetist says sharply before handing him a compress.

The surgeons now begin the long task of sewing: they work to reconnect the heart, moving from bottom to top, anchoring it at four points – the recipient's left atrium is sewn to the corresponding part of the left atrium of the donor's heart, same for the right atrium, the recipient's pulmonary artery is lined up with the donor's right ventricular outflow tract, the aorta to the left ventricular outflow tract. Virgilio massages the heart at regular intervals, pressing hard with both hands, his wrists disappearing inside Claire's body.

A more routine rhythm falls into place now, snippets of conversations swell, sometimes a hubbub of O.R. banter, insider jokes. Harfang asks Virgilio about the game with this mix of condescendence and feigned complicity that annoys the Italian: so, Virgilio, what do you think about the Italians' strategy, do you think it makes for a good game? And the young man replies shortly that Pirlo is an incredible player. The body is operated on in a state of hypothermia, but it's hot now in this O.R., they sponge the physicians' foreheads, temples and lips, they help them to change clothes and gloves regularly – the nurse unseals packages and holds the gowns out flat and inside out. The human energy expended there, the physical tension but also the dynamics of the action – nothing less than a transfer of life – couldn't help but produce this cloud of moisture that begins to form, to hover in the room.

The work of suturing is finally complete. They flush out the organ, evacuate the air in order to prevent bubbles from rising to Claire's brain: the heart can now receive the blood.

The tension spikes again around the table, Harfang says: okay, we're ready, we can start the flow. Now is the moment. The filling happens by the millilitre, requiring a highly calibrated flow – too sudden and the heart could deform and never go back to its original shape – the nurses hold their breath, the anaesthetists are on the alert, the perfusionist is sweating too; only Alice remains imperturbable. No one moves in the O.R., a compact silence covers the operating table as the heart is slowly irrigated. Then comes the electric moment:

Virgilio picks up the defibrillator paddles, holds them out to Harfang, they remain aloft long enough for their eyes to meet and then Harfang nudges his chin in Virgilio's direction, go ahead, you do it – and maybe in that moment Virgilio gathers up all he knows of prayer and superstition, maybe he pleads with Heaven, or, on the contrary, maybe he takes hold of everything that has just been accomplished, the sum of actions and the sum of words, the sum of spaces and emotions – and he carefully places the electric paddles on either side of the heart, casts a glance at the electrocardiogram screen. Everyone clear? Shock! The heart receives the shot, the whole world stands still above what is now Claire's heart. The organ stirs faintly, two, three spasms, then goes still. Virgilio swallows, Harfang has placed his hands on the edge of the bed and Alice is so white that the anaesthetist, scared she might collapse, pulls on her arm so she'll come down from the platform. Second try. Clear?

– Shock!

The heart contracts, a shudder, then moves with nearly imperceptible tremors, but if you come closer, you can see a faint beating, and bit by bit the organ begins to pump blood through the body, and it takes its place again, then the pulsations become regular, strangely rapid, soon forming a rhythm, and their beating is like that of an embryo heart, this twitching that's perceivable from the first ultrasound; and yes, it is the first heartbeat that can be heard, the very first heartbeat, the one that signifies a new beginning.

Did Claire hear Thomas Remige's song during her anaesthetised dreams, this song of a good death? Did she hear his voice in the dark, at four in the morning, when she was receiving Simon Limbeau's heart? She's placed on extracorporeal life support for another half hour, and then she too is sewn up again, retractors releasing the tissue for a delicate damsel's suture, and she remains under surveillance in the O.R., surrounded by black screens that show the luminescent waves of her heart, long enough for her body to recuperate, long enough for the crazy state of the room to be tidied, long enough for them to count the instruments and compresses, for them to wipe up the blood, long enough for the team to break up, and for each one to take off their O.R. clothes and get dressed again, to splash water on their faces and wash their hands, then leave the hospital to go catch the first Metro, long enough for Alice to regain her colour and venture a smile while Harfang whispers in her ear, so, little Harfanguette, what do you think of all this?, long enough for Virgilio to push back his sterile cap and pull down his mask, to decide to ask Alice to go have a beer near Montparnasse, a plate of fries, a rare steak, that old story of prolonging the moment, long enough for her to pull on her white coat again and for him to caress the animal collar, and long enough, finally, for the underbrush to grow light, for the mosses to go blue, for the goldfinch to sing and for the great wave to come to an end in the digital night. It's five forty-nine.

TRANSLATOR'S NOTE

I ended up in the south of France again this past winter, in Arles, at the residency dedicated to literary translators where I first worked on Maylis de Kerangal's novel *Naissance d'un pont* (*Birth of a Bridge*). The residency is housed in the old hospital where Van Gogh was admitted at various points in his difficult life. Between stays, he painted the garden: a square plot enclosed in a stone courtyard, divided neatly into geometrical sections, dominated by the colour yellow and converging at a central fountain where there once were fish. Each day that I grappled with Maylis's labyrinthine phrases, I walked through this garden, and each day I experienced a kind of doubling of consciousness. I breathed in the present-day scents of earth and irises in bloom, simultaneously feeling like I was walking in Van Gogh's painting, "La Cour de l'hôpital d'Arles", from 1889. This seemed to echo the doubling of mind I was experiencing as I translated this book – thinking, sensing, in two languages, with the English sentences like a transparency lain over the original.

Like *Birth of a Bridge*, this book pulls us into the streaming realm of long sentences and what Maylis has called a "language hold-up" (*braquage du langage*) – an inventive use of rare words and concrete vocabularies. Her way is to approach the very tactile, grounded aspects of life in prose that astounds or makes strange, shimmering, beautiful.

Here again, as in *Birth of a Bridge*, character names contain a plethora of references and significance. In my recent conversation with Maylis for *Bomb Magazine*, I learned that she cannot begin writing a book until she knows the character names. She describes names as little stones within a sentence – they remain unchanged, but illuminate the words around them. Birds, flight, tragedy and fixity are themes in the cast of names for *Mend the Living*. *Révol* contains "*vol*" (flight), revolt and revolution – the revolution of 1959, the character's birth year; *Rémige* is a flight feather; *Harfang* is a male snowy owl; and Cordelia *Owl's* last name needs no explanation. *Cordelia* is also reminiscent of King Lear's daughter, linking her to tragedy and the heart. Marthe *Carrare* reminds us of the marble of antiquity and thus again of tragedy. *Marianne* evokes the Mariana Trench (*la Fosse de Marianne*), that bottomless chasm. *Juliette* is another clear link to tragedy and to love. And then there's Simon. Simon's last name in the French book is *Limbres*, which is one letter away from the French word for limbo – *les limbes* – and is also very near to the word for darkness and shadows – *l'ombre*. These echoes would almost certainly have been lost for an Anglophone audience, so I chose to 'translate' this central name. My deep thanks to David Gressot for first suggesting and helping me arrive at Limbeau.

Anyone who spoke to me during the translation of this book knew that I grew obsessed with the "digital night" of the penultimate sentence: "*le temps que . . . s'achève le grand surf dans la nuit digitale.*" What did Maylis have in mind, what image did she intend to project with this enigmatic descriptor, "*digitale*"? And how to approach the fact that French has two distinct words where English has only one – "digital" means both "of or relating to fingers or toes" (*digitale*) and "using or characterized by computer technology" (*numérique*). From talking with her, I know that there were archaeological layers of meaning Maylis wished to express with these few words. She was thinking of the trace writing leaves behind, the trace of this book and the heart transplant described within; night as a kind of screen (but not a computer screen) on which you might press the tips of your digits, leaving behind tactual prints. A gesture towards memory and the act of writing. As I searched for a way to convey all these intentions, I combed through words that express the "digits" aspect of "digital" (words like metacarpal, phalangeal, manual, manipulate). I spoke to Francophone friends about how much the sense of "digital" (as related to computers) was in their hearing of "*digitale*" – a fair bit, they said (it seemed it might not be so distinct from "*numérique*" after all). When I found the word "dactylic" I thought I had struck gold – a word that relates to fingers but also to literature! – but I quickly discarded it, not least because it was making people think of flying dinosaurs. More than one person suggested that what was important was translating what the reader would get, as opposed to the mostly invisible strata of meaning in the author's mind (should one "be true" to the author or to the text?). After a long circuitous journey, I arrived back at "digital," in the original sense of the word, because it's softer, and because it echoes the digitalis of the foxgloves, the homeopathic cure for a weak heart.

At some point while I was in France, during the wandering year I spent working on this translation, a friend sent me a mid-fever revelation he'd had: *art is home*. And I realized that *Réparer les vivants* was the closest thing I'd had to a home in months. All my stuff was in storage. This book was where I spent my time. This book was my constant. On quays and couches in Arles, on mountain paths in Banff, on buses and trains I lived inside these sentences. And in all the places this book took me, there were people who helped me find an expression or solve a linguistic dilemma. Huge thanks to David once again, whose love for this author's work remains steadfast and inspiring; thank you to Dominique for many consultations, to Julie, Valérie, Hélène, and all the other translators and staff at the C.I.T.L.; to Anglophone friends, my mum and Erin in particular, for puzzling out all things digital and phalangeal with me, and to my sister Breanna for consults on what the kids these days are saying; to Alayna for the lake house; thanks to the Banff group, especially to Katie for encouraging me to take measured risks and to Maryse for helping decode; thank you to Nadia and the editors and *Brick Magazine*, and to Mónica and editors at *Bomb Magazine* in New York. My gratitude to the team at Talonbooks in Vancouver, and to everyone at Maclehose Press. This book, my home for a time, becomes a new work as it, like Simon Limbeau's heart, "migrates over the orbs, along the rails, along the roads," reaching this other language. May it bring great richness.

JESSICA MOORE

MAYLIS DE KERANGAL is the author of several novels and short stories. *Naissance d'un pont*, translated here as *Birth of a Bridge*, won both the Prix Franz Hessel and Prix Médicis in 2010. Her fifth novel, *Réparer les vivants* was published in 2014 and won the Grand Prix RTL-Lire and the Student Choice Novel of the Year from France Culture and Télérama. She lives in Paris.

JESSICA MOORE is an author and translator. She is a former Lannan writer-in-residence and winner of a PEN America Translation Award for her translation of *Turkana Boy* by Jean-François Beauchemin. Her first collection of poetry *Everything, Now,* was published in 2012, and her debut album, *Beautiful in Red,* was released in 2013. She lives in Toronto.